Companion Pocketbo

BDC

HUMAN
ANATOMY

Upper Limb and Thorax

Volume 1

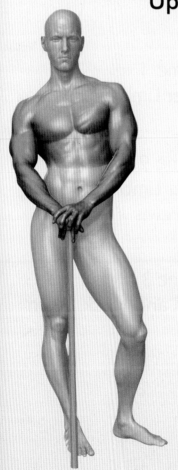

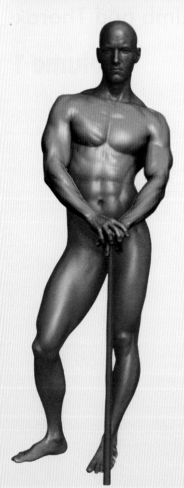

B D Chaurasia's
HUMAN ANATOMY

Upper Limb and Thorax

Volume 1

Edited by

Krishna Garg
MBBS MS PhD FIMSA FIAMS FAMS

Ex-Professor and Head
Department of Anatomy
Lady Hardinge Medical College
New Delhi

CBS

CBS Publishers & Distributors Pvt Ltd

New Delhi • Bengaluru • Pune • Kochi • Chennai

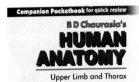

ISBN: 978-81-239-2097-9

Copyright © Editor and Publisher

First Edition: 2012

Published by Satish Kumar Jain and produced by Vinod K. Jain for
CBS Publishers & Distributors Pvt Ltd
4819/XI Prahlad Street, 24 Ansari Road, Daryaganj
New Delhi 110 002, India.   Website: www.cbspd.com
Ph: 23289259, 23266861, 23266867   e-mail: delhi@cbspd.com
Fax: 011-23243014   cbspubs@airtelmail.in

Branches

- Bengaluru: Seema House 2975, 17th Cross, K.R. Road,
  Banasankari 2nd Stage, Bengaluru 560 070, Karnataka
  Ph: +91-80-26771678/79   Fax: +91-80-26771680   e-mail: bangalore@cbspd.com

- Pune: Bhuruk Prestige, Sr. No. 52/12/2+1+3/2 Narhe, Haveli
  (Near Katraj-Dehu Road Bypass), Pune 411 041, Maharashtra
  Ph: 020-64704058, 64704059, 32392277 Fax: +91-020-24300160 e-mail: pune@cbspd.com

- Kochi: 36/14 Kalluvilakam, Lissie Hospital Road, Kochi 682 018,
  Kerala
  Ph: +91-484-4059061-65   Fax: +91-484-4059065   e-mail: cochin@cbspd.com

- Chennai: 20, West Park Road, Shenoy Nagar, Chennai 600 030
  Tamil Nadu
  Ph: +91-44-26260666, 26208620   Fax: +91-44-45530020   email: chennai@cbspd.com

Printed at Manipal Technologies Ltd., Manipal

Preface

<u>BD Chaurasia's *Human Anatomy*</u> has been doing well for a few decades. The three volumes have steadily been enlarging to accommodate gross anatomy, histology, embryology and detailed clinical anatomy. Numerous colour line diagrams support the text of gross, surface and clinical anatomy. Because of its size, it is difficult for the students to revise the volumes prior to their class tests and examinations. This gave us the idea of bringing out a pocketbook based on each volume, giving only "must know" of anatomy. Each pocketbook is almost one-third the size of the main volume containing exclusively the essential components.

The pocketbook is no replacement for the main volume. It is just a complementary book for quick last minute revision of the "volatile anatomy". The illustrations given in the pocketbook are aimed at helping the students review the topics easily as well as retaining and reproducing the information clearly in their examinations. Dissection, clinicoanatomical problems, multiple choice questions, mnemonics, CD containing videos of soft parts and hard parts and questions–answers have not been included in the pocketbook. Knowledge of anatomy and its clinical aspects are provided with equal intensity in the pocketbook. Pocketbook is chiefly meant for first professional undergraduate students. It could be a further help to the students during their clinical postings as they can comfortably keep it in their apron pockets.

Section I on Upper Limb contains tables for muscles of various regions, movements of various joints arteries and branches of nerves are the hallmark of the upper limb section. **Appendix 1** contains nerves of upper limb, arteries of upper limb and clinical terms.

Section II on Thorax contains bones of thoracic cage with its muscles including "respiratory movements". Pleura, lung, bronchial tree, pericardium, heart chambers with their blood supply and nerve supply including clinical anatomy are described briefly. **Appendix 2** contains introduction to autonomic nervous system, blood vessels of thorax in tabulated form and clinical terms.

I am highly obliged to Prof Ved Prakash, Prof Mohini Kaul, Prof Indira Bahl, Prof NA Faruqi, Prof SN Kazi, Prof Suvira Gupta,

Dr Kiran Vasudeva, Dr PS Mittal, Dr Neeraj Master, Dr Azmi Mohsin, Ms Surbhi Garg and other colleagues for sharing their wealth of knowledge and experience.

Ms Nishi Verma and Chand S Naagar of Limited Colors have done the pocketbook with lot of devotion and dedication, under the guidance of Mr YN Arjuna and their staff Mr PS Ghuman and Ms Ritu Chawla of CBS.

Encouragement and support provided by Mr SK Jain, Chairman, CBS, is deeply appreciated. In spite of best efforts, some errors might have crept in while making up the pocketbook. Readers are welcome to point out the shortcomings which will be taken care in its subsequent editions.

Krishna Garg

dr.krishnagarg@gmail.com

Contents

Preface   v

Section I: Upper Limb

1. Introduction   3
2. Bones of Upper Limb   5
3. Pectoral Region   19
4. Axilla   26
5. Back   32
6. Dermatomes and Superficial Veins   35
7. Scapular Region   40
8. Arm   46
9. Forearm and Hand   52
10. Joints of Upper Limb   68
11. Surface Marking   82

     Appendix 1   *85*

Section II: Thorax

12. Introduction   101
13. Bones and Joints of Thorax   105
14. Wall of Thorax   118
15. Thoracic Cavity and the Pleura   121
16. Lungs   125
17. Mediastinum   132
18. Pericardium and Heart   136
19. Superior Vena Cava, Aorta and Pulmonary Trunk   148
20. Trachea, Oesophagus and Thoracic Duct   151
21. Surface Marking of Thorax   155

     Appendix 2   *157*

     Index   *169*

Section I
Upper Limb

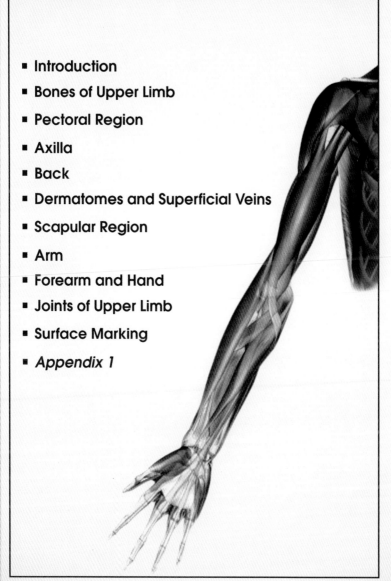

- **Introduction**
- **Bones of Upper Limb**
- **Pectoral Region**
- **Axilla**
- **Back**
- **Dermatomes and Superficial Veins**
- **Scapular Region**
- **Arm**
- **Forearm and Hand**
- **Joints of Upper Limb**
- **Surface Marking**
- *Appendix 1*

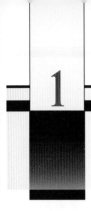

1

Introduction

The fore and hind limbs were evolved basically for bearing the weight of the body and for locomotion. In human body, lower limbs bear the body weight while upper limbs are free to move and to feed oneself.

Each limb is made up of a basal segment or girdle, and a free part divided into proximal, middle and distal segments. The girdle attaches the limb to the axial skeleton. The distal segment carries the five digits.

PARTS OF THE UPPER LIMB

It has been seen that the upper limb is made up of four parts: (1) Shoulder region; (2) arm or brachium; (3) forearm or antebrachium; and (4) hand or manus. Further subdivisions of these parts are given in Table 1.1 and Fig. 1.1.

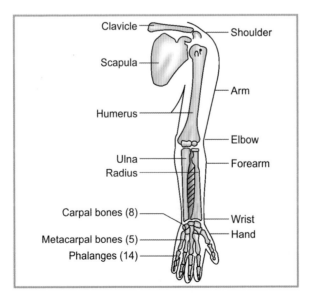

Fig. 1.1: Parts of the upper limb.

Table 1.1: Parts of the upper limb

Parts	Subdivision	Bones	Joints
A. Shoulder region	1. Pectoral region on the front of the chest 2. Axilla or armpit 3. Scapular region on the back	Bones of the shoulder gridle (a) Clavicle (b) Scapula	• Sternoclavicular joint • Acromioclavicular joint
B. Upper arm (arm or brachium) from shoulder to the elbow	—	Humerus (scapulohumeral joint)	Shoulder joint
C. Forearm (antebrachium) from elbow to the wrist	—	(a) Radius (b) Ulna	• Elbow joint • Radioulnar joints
D. Hand	1. Wrist	(a) Carpus, made up of 8 carpal bones	• Wrist joint (radiocarpal joint) • Intercarpal joints
	2. Hand proper	(b) Metacarpus, made up of 5 metacarpal bones	• Carpometacarpal joints
	3. Five digits, numbered from lateral to medial side First Thumb or pollex Second Index or forefinger Third Middle finger Fourth Ring finger Fifth Little finger	(c) 14 phalanges—two for the thumb, and three for each of the four fingers	• Intermetacarpal joints • Metacarpophalangeal joints • Proximal and distal interphalangeal joints

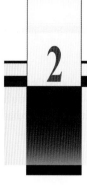

Bones of Upper Limb

CLAVICLE

The clavicle is a long bone (Fig. 2.1). It supports the shoulder so that the arm can swing clearly away from the trunk. The clavicle transmits the weight of the limb to the sternum. The bone has a cylindrical part called the shaft, and two ends, lateral and medial.

Side Determination

The side to which a clavicle belongs can be determined from the following characters.
1. The lateral end is flat. The medial end is large and quadrilateral.
2. The shaft is slightly curved, so that it is convex forwards in its medial two-thirds, and concave forwards in its lateral one-third.
3. The inferior surface is grooved longitudinally in its middle one-third.

Peculiarities of the Clavicle

1. It is the only long bone that lies horizontally
2. It is subcutaneous throughout
3. It is the first bone to start ossifying

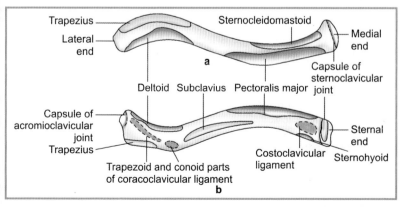

Fig. 2.1: Right clavicle: (a) Superior aspect, (b) Inferior aspect.

4. It is the only long bone which ossifies in membrane
5. It is the only long bone which has two primary centres of ossification

It receives weight of upper limb via lateral one-third through coracoclavicular ligament and transmits it to the axial skeleton via medial two-thirds part through sternoclavicular joint.

Particular Features

Muscles Attached with their Nerve Supply

1. Sternocleidomastoid: Spinal root of accessory nerve
2. Pectoralis major: Medial and lateral pectoral nerves
3. Deltoid: Axillary nerve
4. Trapezius: Spinal root of XI nerve
5. Subclavius: Nerve to subclavius

Ligaments Attached

1. Medial end: Sternoclavicular and costoclavicular
2. Lateral end: Acromioclavicular and coracoclavicular

SCAPULA

The scapula is a thin bone placed on the posterolateral aspect of the thoracic cage. The scapula has two surfaces, three borders, three angles, and three processes (Fig. 2.2).

Three borders: Lateral, medial and superior

Three angles: Superior, inferior and lateral. Lateral angle is surmounted by glenoid cavity.

Three fossae: Supraspinous, infraspinous and subscapularis

Three projections: Spine of scapula, acromion and coracoid process

Side Determination

1. The lateral or glenoid angle is large and bears the glenoid cavity.
2. The dorsal surface is convex and is divided by the triangular spine into the supraspinous and infraspinous fossae. The costal surface is concave to fit on the convex chest wall.
3. The thickest lateral border runs from the glenoid cavity above to the inferior angle below.

Particular Features

Muscles Attached with their Nerve Supply

Borders
Lateral border
• *Long head of triceps brachii:* Radial nerve

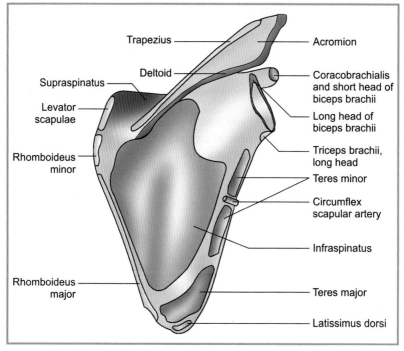

Fig. 2.2: Right Scapula: Dorsal aspect.

- *Teres minor (2 slips):* Axillary nerve
- *Teres major:* Lower subscapular nerve
- *Latissimus dorsi:* Thoracodorsal nerve

Medial border

    (i) *Dorsal surface*

        - *Levator scapulae:* Dorsal scapular nerve (C5)
        - *Rhomboideus minor:* Dorsal scapular nerve (C5)
        - *Rhomboideus major:* Dorsal scapular nerve (C5)

    (ii) *Costal surface:* Three digitations of serratus anterior—long thoracic nerve (C6, C7, C8)

Superior border

Inferior belly of omohyoid—ansa cervicalis (C2, C3)

    Angles

    (i) *Inferior:* Latissimus dorsi on dorsal surface—thoracodorsal nerve. Serratus anterior on costal surface (five digitations)

    (ii) *Superior:* Covered by trapezius

    (iii) *Lateral:* Carries glenoid cavity

    Fossae

    (i) *Supraspinous:* Supraspinatus—suprascapular nerve (C5, C6)

(ii) *Infraspinous:* Infraspinatus—suprascapular nerve (C5, C6)
(iii) *Subscapularis:* Subscapularis—upper and lower subscapular nerves (C5, C6)

Processes
Coracoid Process
Muscles
* *Pectoralis minor:* Medial and lateral pectoral nerves
* *Short head of biceps brachii:* Musculocutaneous nerve
* *Coracobrachialis:* Musculocutaneous nerve

Ligaments
* Coracoacromial
* Coracoclavicular
* Coracohumeral

Spine of scapula and acromion process
* *Deltoid:* Axillary nerve (C5, C6)
* *Trapezius:* Spinal root of XI nerve
* *Supraglenoid tubercle:* Long head of biceps brachii—musculo-cutaneous nerve

HUMERUS

General Features

The humerus is the bone of the arm. It is the longest bone of the upper limb.

Humerus is known as "funny bone" as there is a peculiar sensation when posterior part of medial epicondyle gets hit.

Humerus is a long bone having an upper end, shaft and a lower end.

Upper end comprises head, anatomical neck, greater tubercle intertubercular sulcus, lesser tubercle and surgical neck.

Shaft comprises
Three borders: Anterior, medial and lateral
Three surfaces: Medial, lateral and posterior

Side Determination

1. The upper end is rounded to form the head. The lower end is expanded from side to side and flattened from before backwards.
2. The head is directed medially and backwards.
3. The lesser tubercle projects from the front of the upper end and is limited laterally by the intertubercular sulcus or bicipital groove.

Head Forms Shoulder Joint
Lesser tubercle: Subscapularis—upper and lower subscapular nerves.

Greater Tubercle

Supraspinatus
Infraspinatus   ] Suprascapular nerve

Teres minor: axillary nerve

Intertubercular sulcus: Tendon of long head of biceps brachii passes through this sulcus.

Anatomical neck: Capsule of the shoulder joint is attached here. Its attachment is lower on the medial side to permit abduction of the shoulder joint.

Surgical neck: Axillary nerve and posterior circumflex humeral vessels curves around the surgical neck.

Shaft of Humerus

Anterolateral surface carries deltoid tuberosity in its middle to which deltoid muscle is inserted—axillary nerve.

Anteromedial surface and anterolateral surface in lower halves: Brachialis—musculocutaneous nerve.

Posterior surface: Lateral head of triceps brachii muscle above and big medial head below: In between the two heads lies radial nerve and profunda brachii vessels (Fig. 2.3).

Medial border: Its middle gives attachment of coracobrachialis muscle.

Lateral border in lower part is called lateral supracondylar ridge. It gives attachment to

Brachioradialis from upper two-thirds—radial nerve

Extensor carpi radialis longus from lower one-third—radial nerve

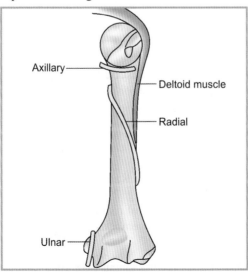

Fig. 2.3: Relation of axillary, radial and ulnar nerves to the back of humerus.

Medial border in lower part is called medial supracondylar ridge and gives attachment to pronator teres—median nerve.

Lower End

It comprises articular capitulum, trochlea and non-articular medial epicondyle and lateral epicondyle.

Lower end also shows radial fossa, coronoid fossa on front and olecranon fossa on the back of humerus.

Medial epicondyle: Origin to superficial flexor muscles of forearm.

Ulnar nerve lies behind this epicondyle (Fig. 2.3).

Lateral epicondyle: Origin to superficial extensor muscles of forearm.

RADIUS

The radius is the lateral bone of the forearm, and is homologous with the tibia of the lower limb.

Radius has an upper end, shaft and a lower end.

Side Determination

The smaller circular upper end is concave followed by a constricted neck. Just below the medial aspect of neck is the radial tuberosity.

The wider lower end is thick with a pointed styloid process on its lateral aspect and a prominent dorsal tubercle on its posterior surface. Medial or interosseous border is thin and sharp.

General Features

Upper End

1. *Head:* Articulates with capitulum of humerus. Its circumference forms superior radioulnar joint.
2. *Neck:* Narrow part
3. *Tuberosity:* Biceps brachii inserted into rough posterior part—Musculocutaneous nerve. Anterior part is covered by a bursa.

Shaft

Shaft has three borders and three surface.

Borders

1. *Anterior border* is oblique. Radial head of flexor digitorum superficialis—median nerve (Fig. 2.4).
2. *Posterior border:* On the back of radius
3. *Medial border:* Interosseous membrane is attached

Surfaces

1. *Anterior surface:* Flexor pollicis longus from upper two-thirds—anterior interosseous nerve.

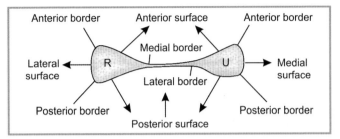

Fig. 2.4: The radius and ulna of right side (on section).

Pronator quadratus inserted into lower one-fourth—anterior interosseous nerve

2. *Lateral surface:* Supinator in upper part—posterior interosseous nerve. Pronator teres in middle part—median nerve
   Brachioradialis in lowest part—radial nerve
3. *Posterior surface:* Abductor pollicis longus and extensor pollicis brevis attached—posterior interosseous nerve.

Lower End

It is the widest part of the radius and has five surfaces

1. *Anterior surface:* Radial artery is felt as radial pulse on the lateral aspect of this surface
2. *Posterior surface:* Shows four grooves for the extensor tendons. Dorsal tubercle lies lateral to an oblique groove
3. *Medial surface* called as ulnar notch for head of ulna
4. *Lateral surface* prolonged as styloid process
5. *Inferior surface* articulates with scaphoid laterally and lunate medially. This surface forms the wrist joint

ULNA

The ulna is the medial bone of the forearm. It presents upper end, shaft and a lower end.

Upper End

Upper end presents beak-like olecranon process, coronoid process, and the trochlear and radial notches.

Shaft

Comprises three borders: Lateral, anterior and posterior
Three surfaces: Anterior, medial and posterior

Lower End

Composed of head and styloid process

Side Determination

1. The upper end is hook-like, with its concavity directed forwards.
2. The lateral border of the shaft is sharp and crest-like.
3. Pointed styloid process lies medial to the rounded head of ulna.

Processes

1. *Olecranon process:* Its superior surface gives insertion to triceps brachii—radial nerve.
   Lateral aspect of olecranon gives insertion to anconeus—radial nerve
2. *Coronoid process:* Its anterior surface gives insertion to brachialis—musculocutaneous nerve.
   Lateral surface of coronoid process gives origin to supinator—posterior interosseous.

Surfaces

1. Anterior and medial surfaces of the shaft in upper three-fourths area gives origin to flexor digitorum profundus muscle—lateral half by anterior interosseous nerve and medial half by ulnar nerve.
2. Lower part of anterior surface gives origin to pronator quadratus—anterior interosseous nerve.
3. Posterior surface gives origin to abductor pollicis longus, extensor pollicis brevis and extensor indicis.
   Nerve supply of all three muscles is posterior interosseous nerve.

CARPAL BONES

The carpus is made up of 8 carpal bones, which are arranged in two rows (Fig. 2.5).

1. *The proximal row contains (from lateral to medial side)*
   (i) Scaphoid,   (ii) lunate,
   (iii) triquetral, and   (iv) pisiform bones
2. *The distal row contains in the same order*
   (i) Trapezium,   (ii) trapezoid,
   (iii) capitate, and   (iv) hamate bones

Identification

1. The *scaphoid* is boat-shaped and has a tubercle on its lateral side
2. The *lunate* is half-moon-shaped or crescentic
3. The *triquetral* is pyramidal in shape and has an isolated oval facet on the distal part of the palmar surface
4. The *pisiform* is pea-shaped and has only one oval facet on the proximal part of its dorsal surface
5. The *trapezium* is quadrangular in shape, and has a crest and a groove anteriorly. It has a concavoconvex articular surface distally

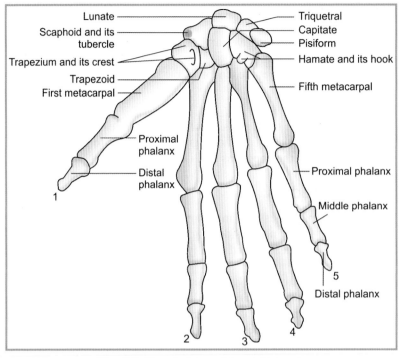

Fig. 2.5: The skeleton of the right hand.

6. The *trapezoid* resembles the shoe of a baby
7. The *capitate* is the largest carpal bone, with a rounded head
8. The *hamate* is wedge-shaped with a hook near its base

Attachments

There are four bony pillars at the four corners of the carpus. All attachments are to these four pillars.

1. The tubercle of the scaphoid gives attachment to
    (i) The flexor retinaculum
    (ii) A few fibres of the abductor pollicis brevis
2. The pisiform gives attachment to
    (i) Flexor carpi ulnaris
    (ii) Flexor retinaculum and its superficial slip
    (iii) Abductor digiti minimi
    (iv) Extensor retinaculum
3. The trapezium has the following attachments
    (i) The crest gives origin to the abductor pollicis brevis, flexor pollicis brevis, and opponens pollicis. These constitute muscles of thenar eminence.

(ii) The edges of the groove give attachment to the two layers of the flexor retinaculum.

(iii) The lateral surface gives attachment to the lateral ligament of the wrist joint.

(iv) The groove lodges the tendon of the flexor carpi radialis—median nerve.

4. Hamate

(i) The tip of the hook gives attachment to the flexor retinaculum

(ii) The medial side of the hook gives attachment to the flexor digiti minimi and the opponens digiti minimi.

METACARPAL BONES

1. The metacarpal bones are 5 miniature long bones, which are numbered from lateral to the medial side (Fig. 2.5).

2. Each bone has a head placed distally, a shaft and a base at the proximal end.

(i) The head is round. It has an articular surface which extends more antero-posteriorly than laterally. It extends more on the palmar surface than on the dorsal surface. The heads of the metacarpal bones form the knuckles.

(ii) The shaft is concave on the palmar surface. Its dorsal surface bears a flat triangular area in its distal part.

(iii) The base is irregularly expanded

Characteristics of Individual Metacarpal Bones

1st   (a) It is the shortest and stoutest of all metacarpal bones.

(b) The base is occupied by a concavo-convex articular surface for the trapezium.

(c) The dorsal surface of the shaft is uniformly convex.

(d) The head is less convex and broader from side to side than the heads of other metacarpals. The ulnar and radial corners of the palmar surface show impressions for sesamoid bones.

(e) The first metacarpal bone is rotated medially through 90° relative to the other metacarpals. As a result of this rotation, the movements of the thumb take place at right angles to those of other digits.

(f) It does not articulate with any other metacarpal bone.

2nd   The base is grooved from before backwards. The medial edge of the groove is larger.

3rd   The base has a styloid process projecting up from the dorsolateral corner.

4th   The base has two small oval facets on its lateral side for the third metacarpal, and on its medial side it has a single elongated facet for the fifth metacarpal.

5th   The base has an elongated articular strip on its lateral side for the fourth metacarpal. The medial side of the base is non-articular and bears a tubercle.

Main Attachments

The main attachment from shaft of metacarpals is of palmar and dorsal interossei muscles. Palmar interossei arise from one bone each except the third metacarpal. Dorsal interossei arise from adjacent sides of two metacarpals.

PHALANGES

There are 14 phalanges in each hand, 3 for each finger and 2 for the thumb. Each phalanx has a base, a shaft and a head.

Attachments

1. *Base of the distal phalanx*
    (a) The *flexor digitorum profundus* is inserted on the palmar surface. Lateral half by anterior interosseous nerve and medial half by ulnar nerve.
    (b) Two side slips of digital expansion fuse to be inserted on the dorsal surface. These also extend the insertion of lumbrical and interossei muscles.
2. *The middle phalanx*
    (a) The *flexor digitorum superficialis* is inserted on each side of the shaft—median nerve
    (b) The fibrous *flexor sheath* is also attached to the side of the shaft.
    (c) A major part of *the extensor digitorum* is inserted on the dorsal surface of the base—posterior interosseous nerve.
3. *The proximal phalanx*
    (a) The fibrous *flexor sheath* is attached to the sides of the shaft.
    (b) On each side of the base, parts of the *lumbricals and interossei* are inserted.
4. In the thumb, the base of the proximal phalanx provides attachments to the following structures.
    (a) The *abductor pollicis brevis* and *flexor pollicis brevis* are inserted on the lateral side–median nerve.
    (b) The *adductor pollicis* and the *first palmar interosseous* are inserted on the medial side both by ulnar nerve.
    (c) The *extensor pollicis brevis* is inserted on the dorsal surface.

5. In the little finger, the medial side of the base of the proximal phalanx provides insertion to the *abductor digiti minimi* and the *flexor digiti minimi–ulnar nerve*.

CLINICAL ANATOMY

- The clavicle is commonly fractured by falling on the outstretched hand (indirect violence). The most common site of fracture is the junction between the two curvatures of the bone, which is the weakest point. The lateral fragment is displaced downwards by the weight of the limb as trapezius muscle alone is unable to support the weight of upper limb.
- The clavicles may be congenitally absent, or imperfectly developed in a disease called *cleidocranial dysostosis*. In this condition, the shoulders droop, and can be approximated anteriorly in front of the chest.
- Paralysis of the serratus anterior causes 'winging' of the scapula. The medial border of the bone becomes unduly prominent, and the arm cannot be abducted beyond 90 degrees.
- The common sites of fracture of humerus are the surgical neck, the shaft, and the supracondylar region.

  Supracondylar fracture is common in young age. It is produced by a fall on the outstretched hand. The lower fragment is mostly displaced backwards, so that the elbow is unduly prominent, as in dislocation of the elbow joint. The three bony points of the flexed elbow form the usual equilateral triangle. This fracture may cause injury to the median nerve. It may also lead to Volkmann's ischaemic contracture caused by occlusion of the brachial artery.
- The humerus has a poor blood supply at the junction of its upper and middle thirds. Fractures at this site show delayed union or non-union.
- The head of the humerus commonly dislocates inferiorly.
- The radius commonly gets fractured about 2 cm above its lower end (Colles' fracture). This fracture is caused by a fall on the outstretched hand. The distal fragment is displaced upwards and backwards, and the radial styloid process comes to lie proximal to the ulnar styloid process. (It normally lies distal to the ulnar styloid process.) If the distal fragment get displaced anteriorly it is called Smith's fracture.
- A sudden powerful jerk on the hand of a child may dislodge the head of the radius from the grip of the annular ligament. This is known as subluxation of the head of the radius (pulled elbow). The head can normally be felt in a hollow behind the lateral epicondyle of the humerus.
- The ulna is the stabilising bone of the forearm, with its trochlear notch gripping the lower end of the humerus. On this foundation the radius can pronate and supinate for efficient working of the upper limb.

- The shaft of the ulna may fracture either alone or along with that of the radius. Cross-union between the radius and ulna must be prevented to preserve pronation and supination of the hand.
- *Dislocation of the elbow* is produced by a fall on the outstretched hand with the elbow slightly flexed. The olecranon shifts posteriorly and the elbow is fixed in slight flexion.

  Normally in an extended elbow, the tip of the olecranon lies in a horizontal line with the two epicondyles of the humerus; and in the flexed elbow the three bony points form an equilateral triangle. These relations are disturbed in dislocation of the elbow.
- *Fracture of the olecranon* is common and is caused by a fall on the point of the elbow. Fracture of the coronoid process is uncommon, and usually accompanies dislocation of the elbow.
- *Madelung's deformity* is dorsal subluxation (displacement) of the lower end of the ulna, due to retarded growth of the lower end of the radius.
- *Fracture of the scaphoid* is quite common. The bone fractures through the waist at right angles to its long axis. The fracture is caused by a fall on the outstretched hand, or on the tips of the fingers. This causes tenderness and swelling in the anatomical snuff box, and pain on longitudinal percussion of the thumb and index finger. The residual disability is more marked in the midcarpal joint than in the wrist joint. The importance of the fracture lies in its liability to non-union, and avascular necrosis of the body of the bone. Normally, the scaphoid has two nutrient arteries, one entering the palmar surface of the tubercle and the other the dorsal surface of the body. Occasionally (13% of cases) both vessels enter through the tubercle or through the distal half of the bone. In such cases, fracture may deprive the proximal half of the bone of its blood supply leading to avascular necrosis.
- Dislocation of the lunate may be produced by a fall on the acutely dorsiflexed hand with the elbow joint flexed. This displaces the lunate anteriorly, also leading to *carpal tunnel syndrome* like features.
- Fracture of the base of the first metacarpal is called Bennett's fracture. It involves the anterior part of the base, and is caused by a force along its long axis. The thumb is forced into a semiflexed position and cannot be opposed. The fist cannot be clenched.
- The other metacarpals may also be fractured by direct or indirect violence. Direct violence usually displaces the fractured segment forwards. Indirect violence displaces them backwards.
- Tubercular or syphilitic disease of the metacarpals or phalanges in a child is located in the middle of the diaphysis rather than in the metaphysis because the nutrient artery breaks up into a plexus immediately upon reaching the medullary cavity. In adults, however,

the chances of infection are minimised because the nutrient artery is replaced (as the major source of supply) by periosteal vessels.

- When the thumb possesses three phalanges, the first metacarpal has two epiphyses one at each end. Occasionally, the first metacarpal bifurcates distally. Then the medial branch has no distal epiphysis, and has only two phalanges. The lateral branch has a distal epiphysis and three phalanges. Total digits are six in such case.

- *Anatomical snuff box* is a triangular depression on the posterolateral aspect of the wrist joint. It is bounded by abductor pollicis longus, extensor pollicis brevis laterally and extensor pollicis longus medially. In its floor are scaphoid and trapezium.

   Radial artery traverses the anatomical snuff box to make its entry into the palm.

   The digital branch of radial nerve pass through it to reach dorsum of hand. Cephalic vein is formed at this box.

   During scaphoid fracture, pain is felt in the anatomical snuff box.

- *Relation of capsular attachments and epiphyseal lines:* If epiphyseal line, i.e. site of union of epiphysis and metaphyseal end of diaphysis is intracapsular, the infection of the joints are likely to affect the metaphysis, the actively growing part of the bone especially in young age.

- Fracture of distal phalanx of middle finger is commonest. It is treated by splinting the injured phalanx to the adjacent normal finger. This is called "buddy splint".

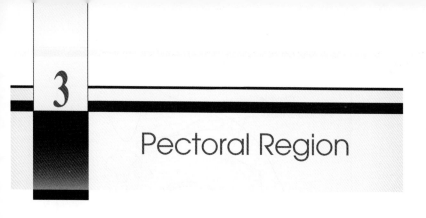

Pectoral Region

BREAST/MAMMARY GLAND

The breast is found in both sexes, but is rudimentary in the male. It is well developed in the female after puberty. The breast is a *modified sweat gland*. It forms an important accessory organ of the female reproductive system, and provides nutrition to the newborn in the form of milk.

Situation

The breast lies in the superficial fascia of the pectoral region. A small extension called the *axillary tail of Spence*, pierces the deep fascia and lies in the axilla.

Extent

(i) Vertically, it extends from the second to the sixth rib.
(ii) Horizontally, it extends from the lateral border of the sternum to the mid-axillary line.

Deep Relations

The deep surface of the breast is related to the parts of three muscles, namely the *pectoralis major,* the *serratus anterior*, and the *external oblique muscle* of the abdomen (Fig. 3.1).

Structure of the Breast

The structure of the breast may be conveniently studied by dividing it into the skin, the parenchyma, and the stroma.

The skin: It covers the gland and presents the following features.

1. A conical projection called the *nipple* is present just below the centre of the breast at the level of the fourth intercostal space. The nipple is pierced by 15 to 20 *lactiferous ducts*.
2. The skin surrounding the base of the nipple is pigmented and forms a circular area called the *areola*.

The parenchyma: It is made up of glandular tissue which secretes milk. The gland consists of 15 to 20 *lobes*.

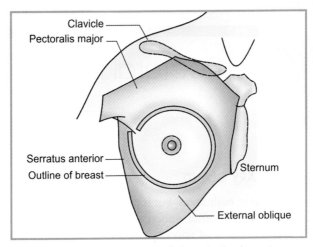

Fig. 3.1: Muscles situated deep to the breast.

The stroma: It forms the supporting framework of the gland. It is partly fibrous and partly fatty.

Blood Supply

The mammary gland is extremely vascular. It is supplied by branches of the following arteries.
1. *Internal thoracic artery* (a branch of the subclavian artery) through its perforating branches
2. The *lateral thoracic,* superior thoracic and acromiothoracic (thoracoacromial) branches of the axillary artery
3. Lateral branches of the *posterior intercostal* arteries.
   The veins follow the arteries.

Nerve Supply

The breast is supplied by the anterior and lateral cutaneous branches of the 4th to 6th intercostal nerves. The nerves do not control the secretion of milk. Secretion is controlled by the hormone *prolactin,* secreted by the pars anterior of the hypophysis cerebri.

Lymphatic Drainage

Lymphatic drainage of the breast assumes great importance to the surgeon because *carcinoma* of the breast spreads mostly along lymphatics to the regional lymph nodes. The subject can be described under two heads, the lymph nodes, and the lymphatics (Fig. 3.2).

Lymph Nodes

Lymph from the breast drains into the following lymph nodes (Fig. 3.2).

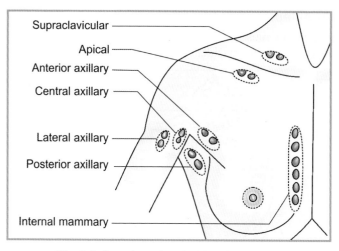

Fig. 3.2: Lymph nodes draining the breast.

1. The axillary lymph nodes, chiefly the *anterior* (or pectoral) group. The *posterior, lateral, central* and *apical* groups of nodes also receive lymph from the breast either directly or indirectly.
2. The *internal mammary* (parasternal) nodes which lie along the internal thoracic vessels.
3. Some lymph from the breast also reaches the *supraclavicular nodes,* the *cephalic* (deltopectoral) node, the *posterior intercostal* nodes (lying in front of the heads of the ribs), the *subdiaphragmatic* and *subperitoneal* lymph plexuses.

Lymphatic Vessels

The *superficial lymphatics* drain the skin over the breast except for the nipple and areola. The lymphatics pass radially to the surrounding lymph nodes (axillary, internal mammary, supraclavicular and cephalic).

The *deep lymphatics* drain the parenchyma of the breast. They also drain the nipple and areola.

Some further points of interest about the lymphatic drainage are as follows.

1. About 75% of the lymph from the breast drains into the *axillary nodes*; 20% into the *internal mammary nodes;* and 5% into the *posterior intercostal nodes.*
2. Lymphatics from the lower and inner quadrants of the breast may communicate with the subdiaphragmatic and subperitoneal lymph plexuses by piercing the anterior abdominal wall. So cancer may spread into the abdominal lymph nodes.

Serratus Anterior

Serratus anterior muscle is not strictly a muscle of the pectoral region, but it is convenient to consider it here (Fig. 3.3).

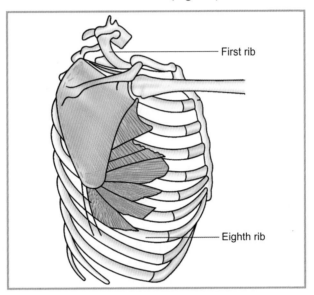

First rib

Eighth rib

Fig. 3.3: Serratus anterior muscle.

Origin

Serratus anterior muscle arises by eight digitations from the upper eight ribs, and from the fascia covering the intervening intercostal muscles.

Insertion

The muscle is inserted into the costal surface of the scapula along its medial border. The first digitation is inserted from the superior angle to the root of the spine.

The next two digitations are inserted lower down on the medial border.

The lower five digitations are inserted into a large triangular area over the inferior angle.

Nerve Supply

The nerve to the serratus anterior is a branch of the brachial plexus. It arises from roots C5, C6 and C7.

Actions

1. Along with the pectoralis minor, the muscle pulls the scapula forwards around the chest wall to protract the upper limb (in pushing and punching movements).

Table 3.1: Muscles of the pectoral region

Muscle	Origin from	Insertion into
Pectoralis major	• Anterior surface of medial half of clavicle • Half the breadth of anterior surface of manubrium and sternum up to sixth costal cartilages • Aponeurosis of the external oblique muscle of abdomen	It is inserted by a bilaminar tendon on the lateral lip of the bicipital groove The two laminae are continuous with each other inferiorly
Pectoralis minor	• 3, 4, 5 ribs, near the costochondral junction • Intervening fascia covering external intercostal muscles	Medial border and upper surface of the coracoid process
Subclavius	First rib at the costochondral junction	Subclavian groove in the middle one-third of the clavicle

Muscle	Nerve supply	Actions

Pectoralis major	Medial and lateral pectoral nerves	• Acting as a whole the muscle causes: Adduction and medial rotation of the shoulder (arm)
		• Clavicular part produces: Flexion of the arm
		• Sternocostal part is used in
		  – Extension of flexed arm against resistance
		  – Climbing

Pectoralis minor	Medial and lateral pectoral nerves	• Draws the scapula forward, (with serratus anterior) • Depresses the point of the shoulder • Helps in forced inspiration
Subclavius	Nerve to subclavius	Steadies the clavicle during movements of the shoulder

2. The fibres inserted into the inferior angle of the scapula pull it forwards and rotate the scapula so that the glenoid cavity is turned upwards. In this action, the serratus anterior is helped by the trapezius which pulls the acromion upwards and backwards.

   When the muscle is paralysed the medial margin of the scapula gets raised specially when 'pushing movements' are attempted. This is called 'winging of the scapula'.

3. The muscle steadies the scapula during weight carrying

4. It helps in forced inspiration

Additional Features

1. Paralysis of the serratus anterior produces 'winging of scapula' in which the inferior angle and the medial border of the scapula are unduly prominent. The patient is unable to do any pushing action, nor can he raise his arm above the head. Any attempt to do these movements makes the inferior angle of the scapula still more prominent.

2. *Clinical testing:* Forward pressure with the hands against a wall, or against resistance offered by the examiner makes the inferior angle of the scapula prominent (winging of scapula) if the serratus anterior is paralysed.

CLINICAL ANATOMY

The breast is a frequent site of carcinoma (cancer). Several anatomical facts are of importance in diagnosis and treatment of this condition. Abscesses may also form in the breast and may require drainage. The following facts are worthy of note.

- Incisions of breast are usually made radially to avoid cutting the lactiferous ducts
- Cancer cells may infiltrate the suspensory ligaments. The breast then becomes fixed. Contraction of the ligaments can cause retraction or puckering (folding) of the skin
- Infiltration of lactiferous ducts and their consequent fibrosis can cause retraction of the nipple
- Obstruction of superficial lymph vessels by cancer cells may produce oedema of the skin giving rise to an appearance like that of the skin of an orange (*peau d' orange* appearance)
- Because of communications of the superficial lymphatics of the breast across the midline, cancer may spread from one breast to the other
- Because of communications of the lymph vessels with those in the abdomen, cancer of the breast may spread to the liver, and cancer cells may 'drop' into the pelvis producing secondaries in the pelvis.

- Apart from the lymphatics, cancer may spread through the segmental veins. In this connection, it is important to know that the veins draining the breast communicate with the vertebral venous plexus of veins. Through these communications cancer can spread to the vertebrae and to the brain.
- Self examination of breasts
  (a) Inspect symmetry of breasts and nipples
  (b) Change in color of skin
  (c) Retraction of nipple is a sign of cancer
  (d) Discharge from nipple on squeezing it
  (e) Palpate all four quadrants with palm of hand. Note any palpable lump
  (f) Raise the arm to feel lymph nodes in axilla
- Mammogram may reveal cancerous mass
- Fine needle aspiration cytology (FNAC) is safe and quick method of diagnosis of lesion of breast
- Retracted nipple is a sign of tumour in the breast
- Size of mammary gland can be increased by putting an implant inside the gland
- Dress designers use their skills to enhance the size of mammary gland. Efforts are made to expose its various quadrants
- Cancer of the mammary gland is the most common cancer in females of all ages. It is more frequently seen in postmenopausal females due to lack of oestrogen hormones
- Self examination of the mammary gland is the only way for early diagnosis and appropriate treatment

4

Axilla

INTRODUCTION

The axilla is the space between upper part of medial side of arm and upper lateral side of thorax. Its shape is pyramidal.

Boundaries

The walls are anterior, posterior, medial and lateral. It has an apex and base.

1. The anterior wall is formed by
   Pectoralis major
   Clavipectoral fascia extending between clavicle and pectoralis minor muscle
   Pectoralis minor
2. The posterior wall is formed by
   Subscapularis
   Latissimus dorsi
   Teres major
3. The medial wall is formed by
   Serratus anterior covering upper part of lateral thoracic wall
4. The lateral wall is narrow and formed by
   Shaft of humerus
   Coracobrachialis
   Short head of biceps brachii
5. Apex is triangular and directed upwards and medially towards root of neck. It is bounded by
   Clavicle anteriorly
   First rib medially
   Upper border of scapula posteriorly
6. Base of axilla is formed by axillary fascia

Contents of the axilla are

(a) The axillary artery and its branches, described in Appendix 1
(b) The axillary vein and its tributaries
(c) The three cords of brachial plexus and their branches (Fig. 4.1)

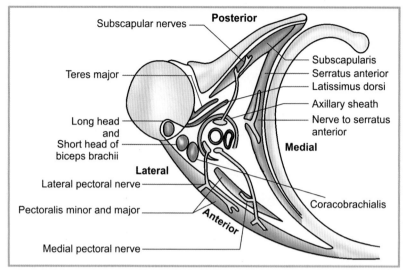

Fig. 4.1: Walls and contents of axilla.

(d) The axillary lymph nodes
(e) Fibrofatty tissue
(f) The axillary tail of Spence of mammary gland in females

BRACHIAL PLEXUS

Brachial plexus is the plexus formed by ventral rami of C5, C6, C7, C8 and T1 nerves. These rami or roots unite, divide, unite again and divide so that most of the muscles get nerve supply from more than one root. Also each branch of brachial plexus gets formed by one, two, three or more roots/rami. So, damage to one root will not cause paralysis of one muscle. These nerve roots carry motor, sensory and sympathetic fibres to the skin and muscles supplied by them. The nerve roots receive sympathetic fibres from middle and inferior cervical and first thoracic ganglia (Fig. 4.2).

A. **Five ventral rami C5, C6, C7, C8 and T1 form brachial plexus**
   Branches from rami
   1. Dorsal scapular or nerve to rhomboideus is given off from C5 for rhomboideus major, rhomboideus minor, responsible for retraction of the scapula and for levator scapulae which elevates the scapula.
   2. Long thoracic from C5, C6, C7 for serratus anterior. Paralysis of the nerve leads to 'winging of scapula' when protraction is attempted.

B. **Ventral rami of C5 and 6 join to form upper trunk**
   Ventral ramus of C7 remains single to form middle trunk
   Ventral rami of C8 and T1 join to form lower trunk

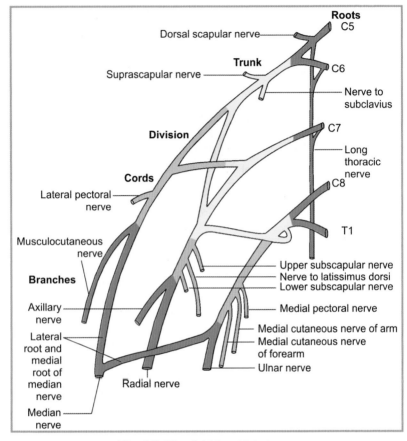

Fig. 4.2: The right brachial plexus.

Branches of upper trunk
1. Suprascapular nerve for supraspinatus and infraspinatus.
2. Nerve to subclavius for subclavius.

C. **Each trunk divides into dorsal and ventral divisions:** Thus there are three ventral divisions for ventral aspect and three dorsal divisions for dorsal aspect of the limb.

D. **and E. cords and their branches:** Ventral divisions of upper and middle trunks join to form lateral cord.

Branches of lateral cord
1. Lateral pectoral nerve for pectoralis major and minor.
2. Musculocutaneous nerve for coracobrachialis, two heads of biceps brachii and brachialis.
3. Lateral root of median nerve joins with its medial root to form median nerve.

Ventral Division of Lower Trunk Remains Single and Forms Medial Cord

Branches of Medial Cord

1. Medial pectoral nerve for pectoralis major and minor
2. Medial cutaneous nerve of arm
3. Medial cutaneous nerve of forearm
4. Medial root of median joins with the lateral root to form median nerve for six and a half muscles of forearm and five muscles of lateral side of palm
5. Ulnar nerve supplies one and a half muscles of forearm and 15 intrinsic muscles of palm

Posterior Cord

Dorsal divisions of upper, middle and lower trunks join together to form *posterior cord.*

Branches of Posterior Cord

1. Upper subscapular for subscapularis, a multipennate muscle
2. Thoracodorsal nerve for latissimus dorsi
3. Lower subscapular for subscapularis and teres major
4. Axillary nerve for deltoid and skin over the lower half of deltoid and teres minor
5. Radial nerve for extensors of elbow, wrist, metacarpophalangeal joints and for supinator

Thus a total of 17 branches are given off from the plexus, including 2 from roots, 2 from trunks, and 13 from cords.

CLINICAL ANATOMY

Injuries to roots, trunks and cords of the brachial plexus may produce characteristic defects, which are described here. Injury to the individual nerves are dealt with each nerve.

Erb's Paralysis

Site of injury: One region of the upper trunk of the brachial plexus is called Erb's point. Six nerves meet here. Injury to the upper trunk causes Erb's paralysis.

Causes of injury: Undue separation of the head from the shoulder, which is commonly encountered in the following:

 (i) Birth injury
 (ii) Fall on the shoulder
(iii) During anaesthesia

   Nerve roots involved: Mainly C5 and partly C6.

Muscles paralysed: Mainly biceps brachii, deltoid, brachialis and brachioradialis. Partly supraspinatus, infraspinatus and supinator.

Deformity (position of the limb)

Arm: Hangs by the side; it is adducted and medially rotated

Forearm: Extended and pronated

The deformity is known as 'policeman's tip hand' or 'porter's tip hand'.

Disability. The following movements are lost

- Abduction and lateral rotation of the arm (shoulder)
- Flexion and supination of the forearm
- Biceps and supinator jerks are lost
- Sensations are lost over a small area over the lower part of the deltoid

Klumpke's Paralysis

Site of injury: Lower trunk of the brachial plexus

Cause of injury: Undue abduction of the arm, as in clutching something with the hands after a fall from a height, or sometimes in birth injury.

Nerve roots involved: Mainly T1 and partly C8.

Muscles paralysed

- Intrinsic muscles of the hand (T1)
- Ulnar flexors of the wrist and fingers (C8)

  Deformity (position of the hand). Claw hand due to the unopposed action of the long flexors and extensors of the fingers. In a claw hand there is hyperextension at the metacarpo-phalangeal joints and flexion at the interphalangeal joints.

Disability

- Claw hand
- Cutaneous anaesthesia and analgesia in a narrow zone along the ulnar border of the forearm and hand.
- *Horner's syndrome:* If T1 is injured proximal to white ramus communicans to first thoracic sympathetic ganglion. There is ptosis, miosis, anhydrosis, enophthalmos, and loss of ciliospinal reflex may be associated. (This is because of injury to sympathetic fibres to the head and neck that leave the spinal cord through nerve T1.)
- *Vasomotor changes:* The skin areas with sensory loss is warmer due to arteriolar dilation. It is also drier due to the absence of sweating as there is loss of sympathetic activity.
- *Trophic changes:* Long-standing case of paralysis leads to dry and scaly skin. The nails crack easily with atrophy of the pulp of fingers.

Injury to the Nerve to Serratus Anterior (Nerve of Bell)

Causes

1. Sudden pressure on the shoulder from above
2. Carrying heavy loads on the shoulder

Deformity: Winging of the scapula, i.e. excessive prominence of the medial border of the scapula. Normally, the pull of the muscle keeps the medial border against the thoracic wall.

Disability

- Loss of pushing and punching actions. During attempts at pushing, there occurs winging of the scapula.
- Arm cannot be raised beyond 90° (i.e. overhead abduction which is performed by the serratus anterior is not possible).

Axilla

- The axilla has abundant axillary hair. Infection of the hair follicles and sebaceous glands gives rise to boils which are common in this area.
- The axillary lymph nodes drain lymph not only from the upper limb but also from the breast and the anterior and posterior body walls above the level of the umbilicus. Therefore, infections or malignant growths in any part of their territory of drainage give rise to involvement of the axillary lymph nodes. Examination of these lymph nodes is, therefore, important in clinical practice. Left axillary nodes to be palpated by right hand. Right axillary nodes have to be palpated by left hand.

  An axillary abscess should be incised through the floor of the axilla, midway between the anterior and posterior axillary folds, and nearer to the medial wall in order to avoid injury to the main vessels running along the anterior, posterior and lateral walls.

- Axillary arterial pulsations can be felt against the lower part of the lateral wall of the axilla.

  In order to check bleeding from the distal part of the limb (in injuries, operations and amputations) the artery can be effectively compressed against the humerus in the lower part of the lateral wall of the axilla.

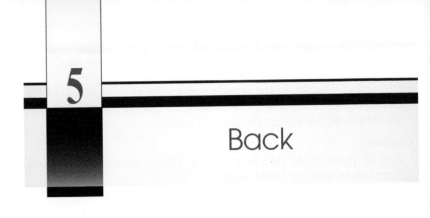

Back

MUSCLES CONNECTING THE UPPER LIMB WITH VERTEBRAL COLUMN

Muscles connecting the upper limb with the vertebral column are the trapezius, the latissimus dorsi, the levator scapulae, and the rhomboideus minor and rhomboideus major. These muscles are described in Tables 5.1 and 5.2.

Structures under Cover of the Trapezius

A large number of structures lie immediately under cover of the trapezius. They are listed below.

Muscles

1. Semispinalis capitis
2. Splenius capitis
3. Levator scapulae
4. Inferior belly of omohyoid
5. Rhomboideus minor
6. Rhomboideus major
7. Supraspinatus
8. Infraspinatus
9. Latissimus dorsi
10. Serratus posterior superior

Vessels

1. Suprascapular artery and vein
2. Superficial branch of the transverse cervical artery
3. Deep branch of transverse cervical artery

Nerves

1. Spinal root of accessory nerve
2. Suprascapular nerve
3. C3, C4 nerves

Bursa

A bursa lies over the smooth triangular area at the root of the spine of the scapula.

Table 5.1: Attachments of muscles connecting the upper limb to the vertebral column

Muscle	Origin from	Insertion into
1. Trapezius The right and left muscles together form a trapezium that covers the upper half of the back	• Medial one-third of superior nuchal line • External occipital protuberance • Ligamentum nuchae • C7 spine • T1–T12 spines • Corresponding supraspinous ligaments	• Upper fibres into the posterior border of lateral one-third of clavicle • Middle fibres, into the medial margin of the acromion and upper lip of the crest of spine of the scapula • Lower fibres, on apex of triangular area at the medial end of the spine.
2. Latissimus dorsi It covers a large area of the lower back, and is overlapped by the trapezius	• Posterior one-third of the outer lip of iliac crest • Posterior layer of lumbar fascia. • Spines of T7–T12 • Lower four ribs • Inferior angle of the scapula	The muscle winds round the lower border of the teres major, and forms the posterior fold of the axilla. The tendon is twisted upside down and is inserted into floor of the intertubercular sulcus
3. Levator scapulae	• Transverse processes of C1, C2 • Posterior tubercles of the transverse processes of C3, C4	Superior angle and upper part of medial border (up to triangular area) of the scapula
4. Rhomboideus minor	• Lower part of ligamentum nuchae • Spines of C7 and T1	Base of the triangular area at the root of the spine of the scapula
5. Rhomboideus major	• Spines of T2, T3, T4, T5 • Supraspinous ligaments	Medial border of scapula below the root of the spine

Table 5.2: Nerve supply and actions of muscles connecting the upper limb to the vertebral column

Muscle	Nerve supply	Actions
Trapezius	• Spinal part of accessory nerve is motor • Branches from C3, C4 are proprioceptive	• Upper fibres act with levator scapulae, and elevate the scapula, as in shrugging • Middle fibres act with rhomboideus, and retract the scapula • Upper and lower fibres act with serratus anterior, and rotate the scapula forwards round the chest wall thus playing an important role in abduction of the arm beyond 90° • Steadies the scapula
Latissimus dorsi	Thoracodorsal nerve (C6, C7, C8) (nerve to latissimus dorsi)	• Adduction, extension, and medial rotation of the shoulder as in swimming, rowing, climbing, pulling, folding the arm behind the back, and scratching the opposite scapula • Helps in violent expiratory effort like coughing, sneezing, etc. • Essentially a climbing muscle • Hold inferior angle of the scapula in place
Levator scapulae	• A branch from dorsal scapular nerve (C5) • C3,C4 branches are proprioceptive	• Helps in elevation of scapula • Steadies the scapula during movements of the arm
Rhomboideus minor	Dorsal scapular nerve (C5)	• Retraction of scapula
Rhomboideus major	Dorsal scapular nerve (C5)	• Retraction of scapula

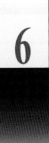

Dermatomes and Superficial Veins

DERMATOMES

DEFINITION

The area of skin supplied by one spinal segment is called a dermatome. A typical dermatome extends from the posterior median line to the anterior median line around the trunk. However, in the limbs the dermatomes have migrated rather irregularly, so that the original uniform pattern is disturbed.

IMPORTANT FEATURES

1. The cutaneous innervation of the upper limb is derived
   (a) Mainly from segments C5–C8 and T1 of the spinal cord, and
   (b) Partly from the overlapping segments from above (C3, C4) as well from below (T2, T3). The additional segments are found only at the proximal end of the limb.

2. The dermatomes of the upper limb are distributed in an orderly numerical sequence.
   (a) Along the preaxial border from above downward, by segments C3–C6
   (b) The middle three digits (index, middle and ring fingers) and the adjoining area of the palm are supplied by segment C7
   (c) The postaxial border is supplied (from below upwards) by segments C8, T1, T2 (Fig. 6.1)

3. As the limb elongates, the central dermatomes (C6–C8) get pulled in such a way that these are represented only in the distal part of the limb, and are buried proximally. The line along which the central dermatomes are buried (missing) while distant dermatomes adjoin each other, and across which the overlapping of the dermatomes is minimal is called the *axial line*. There are two axial lines, ventral and dorsal. The *ventral axial line* extends down almost up to the wrist, whereas the *dorsal axial line* extends only up to the elbow (Fig. 6.1).

35

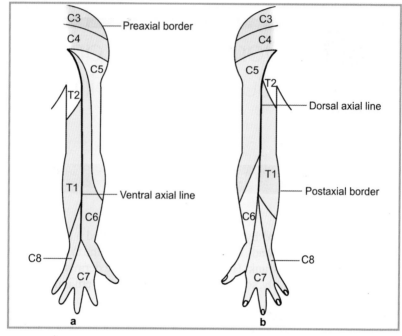

Fig. 6.1: Dermatomes: (a) Anterior aspect, (b) Posterior aspect.

VEINS OF UPPER LIMB

SUPERFICIAL VEINS

Superficial veins of the upper limb assume importance in medical practice because these are most commonly used for intravenous injections for transfusion and for withdrawing blood for testing.

General Remarks

1. Most of the superficial veins of the limb join together to form two large veins, *cephalic* (preaxial) and *basilic* (postaxial).
2. The superficial veins are best utilised for intravenous injections.

INDIVIDUAL VEINS

Dorsal Venous Arch

Dorsal venous arch or dorsal venous plexus lies on the dorsum of the hand. Its afferents (tributaries) include

(i) Three dorsal metacarpal veins.
(ii) A dorsal digital vein from the medial side of the little finger.
(iii) A dorsal digital vein from the radial side of the index finger.

(iv) Two dorsal digital veins from the thumb. The efferents of dorsal venous arch are the cephalic and basilic veins.

Cephalic Vein

Cephalic vein is the preaxial vein of the upper limb. It begins from the lateral end of the dorsal venous arch.

It runs upwards
  (i) Through the roof of the *anatomical snuff box*
  (ii) Winds round the lateral border of the distal part of the forearm
  (iii) Continues upwards in front of the elbow and along the lateral border of the *biceps brachii.*
  (iv) Pierces the deep fascia at the lower border of the pectoralis major
  (v) Runs in the deltopectoral groove up to the infraclavicular fossa
  (vi) It pierces the clavipectoral fascia and joins the axillary vein

At the elbow, the greater part of its blood is drained into the basilic vein through the *median cubital vein,* and partly also into the *deep veins* through the *perforator veins.*

Basilic Vein

Basilic vein is the postaxial vein of the upper limb. It begins from the medial end of the dorsal venous arch.

It runs upwards
  (i) Along the back of the medial border of the forearm
  (ii) Winds round this border near the elbow
  (iii) Continues upwards in front of the elbow (medial epicondyle) and along the medial margin of the biceps brachii up to the middle of the arm where
  (iv) It pierces the deep fascia
  (v) Runs along the medial side of the *brachial artery* up to the lower border of *teres major* where it becomes the axillary vein.

About 2.5 cm above the medial epicondyle of the humerus, it is joined by the median cubital vein.

Median Cubital Vein

Medial cubital vein is a large communicating vein which shunts blood from the cephalic to the basilic vein.

It begins from the cephalic vein 2.5 cm below the bend of the elbow, runs obliquely upward and medially, and ends in the basilic vein 2.5 cm above the medial epicondyle. It is separated from the brachial artery by the *bicipital aponeurosis.*

It is connected to the deep veins through a perforator vein which pierces the bicipital aponeurosis. The perforator vein fixes the median cubital vein and thus makes it ideal for intravenous injections.

Axillary Vein

The *axillary vein* is the continuation of the *basilic vein*. The axillary vein is joined by the *venae comitantes* of the *brachial artery* a little above the lower border of the teres major. It lies on the medial side of the axillary artery. At the outer border of the first rib it becomes the *subclavian vein*.

CLINICAL ANATOMY

- The area of sensory loss of the skin, following injuries of the spinal cord or of the nerve roots, conforms to the dermatomes. Therefore, the segmental level of the damage to the spinal cord can be determined by examining the dermatomes for touch, pain, and temperature. Note that injury to a peripheral nerve produces sensory loss corresponding to the area of distribution of that nerve.
- The spinal segments do not lie opposite to the corresponding vertebrae. In estimating the position of a spinal segment in relation to the surface of the body it is important to remember that a vertebral spine is always *lower* than the corresponding spinal segment. As a rough guide it may be stated that in the cervical region there is a difference of one segment, e.g. the 5th cervical spine overlies the 6th cervical spinal segment.

Spinal segments	Spine of vertebra
$C_1 C_8$	C_1-C_7
T_1-T_6	T_1-T_4
T_7-T_{12}	T_5-T_9
L_1-L_5	$T_{10}-T_{11}$
S_1-S_5 and Co_1	$T_{12}-L_1$

- The median cubital vein is the vein of choice for intravenous injections, for withdrawing blood from donors, and for cardiac catheterisation, because it is fixed by the perforator and does not slip away during piercing. When the median cubital vein is absent, the basilic is preferred over the cephalic because the former is a more efficient channel. Basilic vein runs along straight path, wheras cephalic vein bends acutely to drain into the axillary vein.
- The cephalic vein frequently communicates with the external jugular vein by means of a small vein which crosses in front of the clavicle. In operations for removal of the breast (in carcinoma), the axillary lymph nodes are also removed, and it sometimes becomes necessary to remove a segment of the axillary vein also. In these cases, the

communication between the cephalic vein and the external jugular vein enlarges considerably and helps in draining blood from the upper limb.

In case of fracture of the clavicle, the rupture of the communicating channel may lead to formation of a large haematoma, i.e. collection of blood.

- Inflammation of lymph vessels is known as *lymphangiitis.* In acute lymphangiitis, the vessels may be seen through the skin as red, tender (painful to touch) streaks.
- Inflammation of lymph nodes is called *lymphadenitis.* It may be acute or chronic. The nodes enlarge and become palpable and painful.
- Obstruction to lymph vessels can result in accumulation of tissue fluid in areas of drainage.
  This is called *lymphoedema.* This may be caused by carcinoma, infection with some parasites like filaria, or because of surgical removal of lymph nodes. Filariasis in lower limb leads to increase in its size called as elephantiasis.
- Pain along the medial side of upper arm is due to pressure on the intercostobrachial nerve by enlarged central group of axillary lymph nodes.

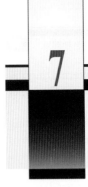

Scapular Region

MUSCLES OF THE SCAPULAR REGION

These are the deltoid: the supraspinatus, the infraspinatus, the teres minor, the subscapularis, and the teres major. The deltoid is described below. The other muscles are described in Table 7.1.

Deltoid

Origin

1. The anterior border of the lateral one-third of the clavicle (Fig. 7.1)
2. The lateral border of the acromion where four septa of origin are attached
3. Lower lip of the crest of the spine of the scapula

Insertion

The deltoid tuberosity of the humerus where three septa of insertion are attached.

Nerve Supply

Axillary nerve (C5, C6)

Structure

The acromial part of deltoid is an example of a multipennate muscle. Many fibres arise from four septa of origin that are attached above to the acromion. The fibres converge on to three septa of insertion which are attached to the deltoid tuberosity. A multipennate arrangement allows a large number of muscle fibres to be packed into a relatively small volume. As the strength of contraction of a muscle is proportional to the number of muscle fibres present in it (and not on their length), a multipennate muscle is much stronger than other muscles having the same volume.

Actions

1. The acromial fibres are powerful abductors of the arm at the shoulder joint from beginning to 90°

Table 7.1: Attachments of muscles of scapular region (except deltoid)

Muscle	Origin from	Insertion into
1. **Supraspinatus**	Medial two-thirds of the supraspinous fossa of the scapula	Upper impression on the greater tubercle of the humerus
2. **Infraspinatus**	Medial two-thirds of the infraspinous fossa of the scapula	Middle impression on the greater tubercle of the humerus
3. **Teres minor**	Upper two-thirds of the dorsal surface of the lateral border of the scapula	Lowest impression on the greater tubercle of the humerus
4. **Subscapularis** (multipennate)	Medial two-thirds of the subscapular fossa	Lesser tubercle of the humerus
5. **Teres major**	Lower one-third of the dorsal surface of lateral border and inferior angle of the scapula	Medial lip of the bicipital groove of the humerus

Muscle	Nerve supply	Actions
1. **Supraspinatus**	Suprascapular nerve (C5, C6)	• Along with other short scapular muscles it steadies the head of the humerus during movements of the arm. Its action as abductor of shoulder joint from 0 to 15° is controversial.
2. **Infraspinatus**	Suprascapular nerve (C5, C6)	• Lateral rotator of arm.
3. **Teres minor**	Axillary nerve (C5, C6)	Same as infraspinatus
4. **Subscapularis**	Upper and lower subscapular nerves (C5, C6)	Medial rotator and adductor of arm
5. **Teres major**	Lower subscapular nerve (C5, C6)	Same as subscapularis

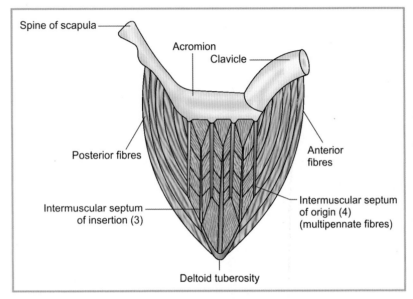

Fig. 7.1: The origin and insertion of the deltoid muscle.

2. The anterior fibres are flexors and medial rotators of the arm
3. The posterior fibres are extensors and lateral rotators of the arm

Structures Under Cover of the Deltoid

Bones

   (i) The upper end of the humerus
  (ii) The coracoid process

Muscles

Insertions of

    (i) Pectoralis minor on coracoid process
   (ii) Supraspinatus, infraspinatus, and teres minor (on the greater tubercle of the humerus)
  (iii) Subscapularis on lesser tubercle of humerus
  (iv) Pectoralis major, teres major and latissimus dorsi on the intertubercular sulcus of the humerus

Origin of

    (i) Coracobrachialis and short head of biceps brachii from the coracoid process
   (ii) Long head of the biceps brachii from the supraglenoid tubercle
  (iii) Long head of the triceps brachii from the infraglenoid tubercle
  (iv) The lateral head of the triceps brachii from the upper part of shaft of the humerus

Vessels

  (i) Anterior circumflex humeral

  (ii) Posterior circumflex humeral

Nerve

Axillary

Joints and Ligaments

  (i) Musculotendinous cuff of the shoulder

  (ii) Coracoacromial ligament

Bursae

All bursae around the shoulder joint, including the subacromial or subdeltoid bursa.

Musculotendinous Cuff of the Shoulder or Rotator Cuff

Musculotendinous cuff of the shoulder is a fibrous sheath formed by the four flattened tendons which blend with the capsule of the shoulder joint and strengthen it. The muscles which form the cuff arise from the scapula and are inserted into the lesser and greater tubercles of the humerus. They are the subscapularis, the supraspinatus, the infraspinatus and the teres minor (Fig. 7.2). Their tendons, while crossing the shoulder joint, become flattened and blend with each other on one hand, and with the capsule of the joint on the other hand, before reaching their points of insertion.

    The cuff gives strength to the capsule of the shoulder joint all around except inferiorly. This explains why dislocations of the humerus occur most commonly in a downward direction.

Intermuscular Spaces

Three intermuscular spaces are to be seen in the scapular region. These are as follows.

Quadrangular Space

Boundaries

  Superior

    (i) Subscapularis in front   (ii) Capsule of the shoulder joint

  (iii) Teres minor behind

  Inferior: Teres major

  Medial: Long head of the triceps brachii

  Lateral: Surgical neck of the humerus

Contents

  (i) Axillary nerve

  (ii) Posterior circumflex humeral vessels

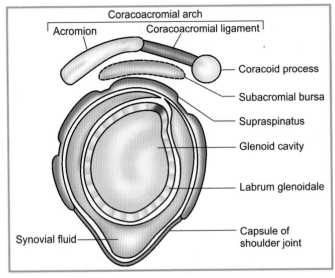

Fig. 7.2: The subacromial bursa as seen in sagittal section.

Upper Triangular Space

Boundaries
   Medial: Teres minor
   Lateral: Long head of the triceps brachii
   Inferior: Teres major

Contents
Circumflex scapular artery. It interrupts the origin of the teres minor and reaches the infraspinous fossa for anastomoses with the suprascapular artery and deep branch of transverse cervical artery.

Lower Triangular Space

Boundaries
   Medial: Long head of the triceps brachii
   Lateral: Medial border of humerus
   Superior: Teres major

Contents
   (i) Radial nerve
   (ii) Profunda brachii vessels

CLINICAL ANATOMY

• Intramuscular injections are often given into the deltoid. They should be given in the middle of the muscle to avoid injury to the axillary nerve.

- In subacromial bursitis, pressure over the deltoid below the acromion with the arm by the side causes pain. However, when the arm is abducted pressure over the same point causes no pain, because the bursa disappears under the acromion (Dawbarn's sign). Subacromial or subdeltoid bursitis is usually secondary to inflammation of the supraspinatus tendon.
- The tendon of the supraspinatus may undergo degeneration. This can give rise to calcification and even spontaneous rupture of the tendon.
- The axillary nerve may be damaged by dislocation of the shoulder or by the fracture of the surgical neck of the humerus. The effects produced are as follows.
    (a) Rounded contour of shoulder is lost; greater tubercle of humerus becomes prominent
    (b) Deltoid is paralysed, with loss of the power of abduction up to 90° at the shoulder
       The deltoid muscle is tested by asking the patient to abduct the arm against resistance applied with one hand, and feeling for the contracting muscle with the other hand
    (c) There is sensory loss over the lower half of the deltoid in a badge like area called regimental badge
- The arterial anastomoses provide a collateral circulation through which blood can flow to the limb when the distal part of the subclavian artery, or the proximal part of the axillary artery is blocked.

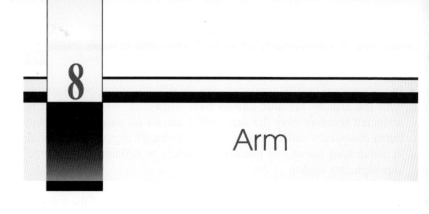

Arm

COMPARTMENTS OF THE ARM

The arm is divided into anterior and posterior compartments by extension of deep fascia which are called the *medial and lateral intermuscular septa.*

ANTERIOR COMPARTMENT

MUSCLES

Muscles of the anterior compartment of the arm are the coracobrachialis, the biceps brachii and the brachialis. They are described in Table 8.1.

Changes at the level of Insertion of Coracobrachialis

1. *Bone*: The circular shaft becomes triangular below this level
2. *Fascial septa*: The medial and lateral intermuscular septa become better defined from this level
3. *Muscles*
    (i) Deltoid and coracobrachialis are inserted at this level
    (ii) Upper end of origin of brachialis extends till this level
    (iii) Upper end of origin of the medial head of triceps brachii extends till here
4. *Arteries*
    (i) The brachial artery passes from the medial side of the arm to its anterior aspect
    (ii) The profunda brachii artery runs in the spiral groove and divides into its anterior and posterior descending branches
    (iii) The superior ulnar collateral artery originates from the brachial artery, and pierces the medial intermuscular septum with the ulnar nerve
    (iv) The nutrient artery of the humerus enters the bone
5. *Veins*
    (i) The basilic vein pierces the deep fascia
    (ii) Two venae comitantes of the brachial artery may unite to form one brachial vein

Table 8.1: Attachments of muscles of arm

Muscle	Origin from	Insertion into
1. Coracobrachialis	• The tip of the coracoid process with the short head of the biceps brachii	The middle 5 cm of the medial border of the humerus
2. Biceps brachii	It has two heads of origin • The short head arises with coracobrachialis from the tip of the coracoid process • The long head arises from the supraglenoid tubercle of the scapula and from the glenoidal labrum. The tendon is intracapsular	• Posterior rough part of the radial tuberosity. The tendon is separated from the anterior part of the tuberosity by a bursa (Fig. 8.1) • The tendon gives off an extension called the bicipital aponeurosis which separates median cubital vein from brachial artery
3. Brachialis	• Lower half of the front of the humerus, including both the anteromedial and anterolateral surfaces and the anterior border Superiorly the origin embraces the insertion of deltoid • Medial and lateral intermuscular septa	• Coronoid process and ulnar tuberosity • Rough anterior surface of the coronoid process of the ulna

Muscle	Nerve supply	Actions
1. Coracobrachialis	Musculocutaneous nerve (C5–C7)	Flexes the arm at the shoulder joint
2. Biceps brachii	Musculocutaneous nerve (C5, C6)	• It is strong supinator when the forearm is flexed All screwing movements are done with it • It is a flexor of the elbow.
3. Brachialis	• Musculocutaneous nerve is motor • Radial nerve is proprioceptive	Flexes forearm at the elbow joint

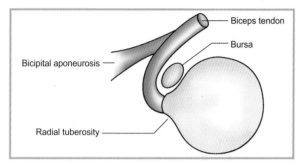

Fig. 8.1: The precise mode of insertion of the biceps brachii muscle.

6. *Nerves*
   (i) The median nerve crosses the brachial artery from the lateral to the medial side
   (ii) The ulnar nerve pierces the medial intermuscular septum with the superior ulnar collateral artery and goes to the posterior compartment
   (iii) The radial nerve pierces the lateral intermuscular septum with the anterior descending (radial collateral) branch of the profunda brachii artery and passes from the posterior to the anterior compartment
   (iv) The medial cutaneous nerve of the arm pierces the deep fascia
   (v) The medial cutaneous nerve of the forearm pierces the deep fascia

MUSCULOCUTANEOUS NERVE   See Appendix 1.

BRACHIAL ARTERY   See Appendix 1.

CUBITAL FOSSA

Cubital fossa is a triangular hollow situated on the front of the elbow. (It is homologous with the popliteal fossa of the lower limb situated on the back of the knee.)

Boundaries

Laterally — Medial border of the brachioradialis
Medially — Lateral border of the pronator teres (Fig. 8.2)
Base   — It is directed upwards, and is represented by an imaginary line joining the front of two epicondyles of the humerus
Apex   — It is directed downwards, and is formed by the meeting point of the lateral and medial boundaries.

Roof

The roof of the cubital fossa is formed by
(a) Skin

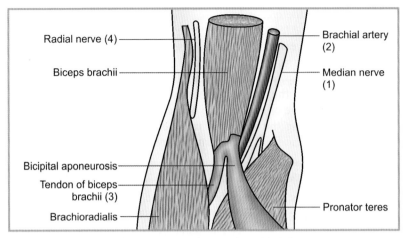

Fig. 8.2: Contents of the right cubital fossa.

(b) Superficial fascia containing the median cubital vein, the lateral cutaneous nerve of the forearm and the medial cutaneous nerve of the
forearm

(c) Deep fascia and (d) Bicipital aponeurosis

Floor

It is formed by
(a) Brachialis and
(b) Supinator muscles

Contents

The fossa is actually very narrow. The contents described are seen after
retracting the boundaries. From medial to the lateral side, the contents
are as follows.

1. The *median nerve*. It gives branches to flexor carpi radialis, palmaris
   longus, flexor digitorum superficialis and leaves the fossa by passing
   between the two heads of pronator teres.
2. The termination of the *brachial artery*, and the beginning of the radial
   and ulnar arteries lie in the fossa. The radial artery is smaller and more
   superficial than the ulnar artery. It gives off the radial recurrent branch.
   The ulnar artery goes deep to both heads of pronator teres and runs
   downwards and medially, being separated from the median nerve by
   the deep head of the pronator teres. It gives off the anterior ulnar
   recurrent, the posterior ulnar recurrent, and the common interosseous
   branches. The common interosseous branch divides into the anterior
   and posterior interosseous arteries, and latter gives off the interosseous
   recurrent branch.

3. The tendon of the *biceps brachii*
4. The *radial nerve* (accompanied by the radial collateral artery) appears in the gap between the brachialis (medially) and the brachioradialis and extensor carpi radialis longus laterally. While running in the intermuscular gap, radial nerve supplies the three flanking muscles. At the level of the lateral epicondyle it gives off the posterior interosseous nerve or deep branch of the radial nerve which leaves the fossa by piercing the supinator muscle. The remaining superficial branch runs in the front of forearm for some distance.

POSTERIOR COMPARTMENT

The region contains the triceps brachii muscle, the radial nerve and the profunda brachii vessels. The nerve and vessels run between the two humeral heads of this muscle. The ulnar nerve runs through the lower part of this compartment.

TRICEPS BRACHII MUSCLE

Origin

Triceps brachii muscle arises by the following three heads
1. The *long head* arises from the infraglenoid tubercle of the scapula; it is the longest of the three heads.
2. The *lateral head* arises from an oblique ridge on the upper part of the posterior surface of the humerus, corresponding to the lateral lip of the radial (spiral) groove.
3. The *medial head* arises from a large triangular area on the posterior surface of the humerus below the radial groove, as well as from the medial and lateral intermuscular septa. At the level of the radial groove, the medial head is medial to the lateral head.

Insertion

The long and lateral heads converge and fuse to form a superficial flattened tendon which covers the medial head and are inserted into the posterior part of the superior surface of the olecranon process of ulna.

Nerve Supply

Each head receives a separate branch from the radial nerve (C7, C8). The branches arise in the axilla and in the radial groove.

Actions

The triceps is a powerful active extensor of the elbow. The long head supports the head of the humerus in the abducted position of the arm. Gravity extends the elbow passively.

RADIAL NERVE See Appendix 1.

CLINICAL ANATOMY

- Brachial pulsations are felt and auscultated in front of the elbow just medial to the tendon of biceps while recording the blood pressure.
- Although the brachial artery can be compressed anywhere along its course, it can be compressed most favourably in the middle of the arm, where it lies on the tendon of the coracobrachialis.
- The cubital region is important for the following reasons
  (a) The median cubital vein is often the vein of choice for intravenous injections
  (b) The blood pressure is universally recorded by auscultating the brachial artery in front of the elbow
- The anatomy of the cubital fossa is useful while dealing with the fracture around the elbow, like the supracondylar fracture of the humerus.
- In radial nerve injuries in the arm, the triceps brachii usually escapes complete paralysis because the nerves supplying it arise in the axilla.
- The radial nerve is very commonly damaged in the region of the radial (spiral) groove. The common causes of injury are as follows.
  (a) Sleeping in an armchair with the limb hanging by the side of the chair (Saturday night palsy), or even by the pressures of the crutch (crutch paralysis)
  (b) Fractures of the shaft of the humerus. This results in the weakness and loss of power of extension at the wrist (wrist drop) and sensory loss over a narrow strip on the back of forearm, and on the lateral side of the dorsum of the hand
- Wrist drop is quite disabling, because the patient cannot grip any object firmly in the hand without the synergistic action of the extensors.

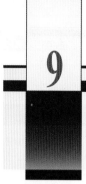

Forearm and Hand

FRONT OF FOREARM

The front of the forearm presents the following components for study.

Components

1. Eight muscles, five superficial and three deep
2. Two arteries, radial and ulnar (see Appendix 1)
3. Three nerves, median, ulnar and radial (see Appendix 1)
   The superficial and deep muscles are shown in Tables 9.1 to 9.4

Flexor Retinaculum

Flexor retinaculum is a strong fibrous band which bridges the anterior concavity of the carpus and converts it into a tunnel, the *carpal tunnel.*

Attachments

Medially, to
1. The pisiform bone (Fig. 9.1)
2. To the hook of the hamate

Laterally, to
1. The tubercle of the scaphoid, and
2. The crest of the trapezium

On either side the retinaculum has a slip
1. The lateral *deep slip* is attached to the medial lip of the groove on the trapezium which is thus converted into a tunnel for the tendon of the flexor carpi radialis;
2. The medial *superficial slip (volar carpal ligament)* is attached to the pisiform bone. The ulnar vessels and nerves pass deep to this slip.

Relations

The structures passing superficial to the flexor retinaculum are
   (i) The palmar cutaneous branch of the median nerve
   (ii) The tendon of the palmaris longus
   (iii) The palmar cutaneous branch of the ulnar nerve

Table 9.1: Attachment of the superficial muscles

Name	Origin	Insertion
1. **Pronator teres**	Medial epicondyle of humerus	Middle of lateral aspect of shaft of radius
2. **Flexor carpi radialis**	Medial epicondyle of humerus	Bases of second and third metacarpal bones
3. **Palmaris longus**	Medial epicondyle of humerus	Flexor retinaculum and palmar aponeurosis
4. **Flexor digitorum superficialis**		
Humeroulnar head	Medial epicondyle of humerus; medial border of coronoid process of ulna	Muscle divides into 4 tendons. Each tendon divides into 2 slips which are inserted on sides of middle phalanx of 2nd to 5th digits
Radial head	Anterior oblique line of shaft of radius	
5. **Flexor carpi ulnaris**		
Humeral head	Medial epicondyle of humerus	Pisiform bone; insertion prolonged to hook of the hamate and base of fifth metacarpal bone
Ulnar head	Posterior border of ulna	

Table 9.2: Attachment of the superficial muscles

Muscle	Nerve Supply	Actions
1. **Pronator teres**	Median nerve	Pronation of forearm
2. **Flexor carpi radialis**	Median nerve	Flexes and abducts hand at wrist joint
3. **Palmaris longus**	Median nerve	Flexes wrist joint
4. **Flexor digitorum superficialis** Humeroulnar and radial heads	Median nerve	Flexes middle phalanx of fingers and assists in flexing proximal phalanx and wrist joint
5. **Flexor carpi ulnaris** Humeral and ulnar heads	Ulnar nerve	Flexes and adducts the hand at the wrist joint

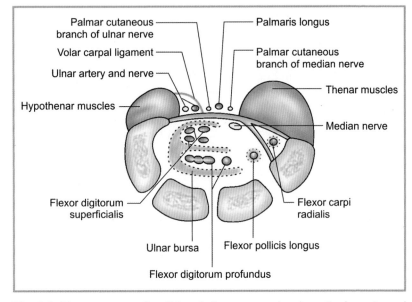

Fig. 9.1: Transverse section through the carpus showing attachments and relations of the flexor retinaculum.

   (iv) The ulnar vessels
   (v) The ulnar nerve. The thenar and hypothenar muscles arise from the retinaculum (Fig. 9.1)

The structures passing deep to the flexor retinaculum are
   (i) The median nerve
  (ii) Four tendons of the flexor digitorum superficialis
 (iii) Four tendons of the flexor digitorum profundus
  (iv) The tendon of the flexor pollicis longus
   (v) The ulnar bursa
  (vi) The radial bursa
 (vii) The tendon of the flexor carpi radialis lies between the retinaculum and its deep slip, in the groove on the trapezium

INTRINSIC MUSCLES OF THE HAND

The intrinsic muscles of the hand serve the function of adjusting the hand during gripping and also for carrying out fine skilled movements. The origin and insertion of these muscles is within the territory of the hand.

There are 20 muscles in the hand, as follows.

1. (a) *Three muscles of thenar eminence*
   (i) Abductor pollicis brevis
  (ii) Flexor pollicis brevis

(iii) Opponens pollicis
(b) *One adductor of thumb:* Adductor pollicis
2. *Four hypothenar muscles*
   (i) Palmaris brevis
  (ii) Abductor digiti minimi
 (iii) Flexor digiti minimi
 (iv) Opponens digiti minimi
   Muscles (ii)–(iv) are muscles of hypothenar eminence
3. *Four lumbricals*
4. *Four palmar interossei*
5. *Four dorsal interossei*
   These muscles are described in Tables 9.5 and 9.6.

SPACES OF THE HAND

The arrangement of fasciae and the fascial septa in the hand is such that many spaces are formed. These spaces are of surgical importance because they may become infected and distended with pus.

A. Palmar spaces
   1. Pulp space of the fingers
   2. Midpalmar space
   3. Thenar space (Table 9.7)
B. Dorsal spaces
   1. Dorsal subcutaneous space
   2. Dorsal subaponeurotic space
C. The forearm space of parona

BACK OF FOREARM AND HAND

Extensor Retinaculum

The deep fascia on the back of the wrist is thickened to form the extensor retinaculum which holds the extensor tendons in place. It is an oblique band, directed downwards and medially. It is about 2 cm broad vertically.

Attachments

Laterally, to the lower part of the *anterior* border of the radius. Medially, to:
   (i) Styloid process of the ulna
  (ii) Triquetral
 (iii) Pisiform

Compartments

The retinaculum sends down septa which are attached to the longitudinal ridges on the posterior surface of the lower end of radius. In this way, 6 osseofascial compartments are formed on the back of the wrist. The

Table 9.3: Attachments of the deep muscles

Muscle	Origin from	Insertion
1. Flexor digitorum profundus (composite or hybrid muscle)	• Upper three-fourths of the anterior and medial surface of the shaft of ulna • Upper three-fourths of the posterior border of ulna • Medial surface of the olecranon and coronoid processes of ulna • Adjoining part of the anterior surface of the interosseous membrane	• The muscle forms 4 tendons for the medial 4 digits which enter the palm by passing deep to the flexor retinaculum • Opposite the proximal phalanx of the corresponding digit the tendon perforates the tendon of the flexor digitorum superficialis • Each tendon is inserted on the palmar surface of the base of the distal phalanx
2. Flexor pollicis longus	• Upper three-fourths of the anterior surface of the shaft of radius • Adjoining part of the anterior surface of the interosseous membrane	• The tendon enters the palm by passing deep to the flexor retinaculum • It is inserted into the palmar surface of the distal phalanx of the thumb
3. Pronator quadratus	Oblique ridge on the lower one-fourth of anterior surface of the shaft of ulna, and the area medial to it	• Superficial fibres into the lower one-fourth of the anterior surface and the anterior border of the radius • Deep fibres into the triangular area above the ulnar notch

Table 9.4: Nerve supply and actions of the deep muscles

Muscle	Nerve Supply	Actions
1. **Flexor digitorum profundus**	• Medial half by ulnar nerve • Lateral half by anterior interosseous nerve (C8, T1)	• Flexor of distal phalanges after the flexor digitorum superficialis has flexed the middle phalanges • Secondarily it flexes the other joints of the digits and fingers, and the wrist • It is the chief gripping muscle. It acts best when the wrist is extended
2. **Flexor pollicis longus**	Anterior interosseous nerve	• Flexes the distal phalanx of the thumb. Continued action may also flex the proximal joints crossed by the tendon
3. **Pronator quadratus**	Anterior interosseous nerve	• Superficial fibres pronate the forearm • Deep fibres bind the lower ends of radius and ulna

Table 9.5: Attachments of small muscles of the hand

Name	Origin	Insertion
Muscles of Thenar eminence		
Abductor pollicis brevis	Tubercle of scaphoid, trapezium, flexor retinaculum	Base of proximal phalanx of thumb (lateral side)
Flexor pollicis brevis	Flexor retinaculum, trapezoid and capitate bones	Base of proximal phalanx of thumb
Opponens pollicis	Flexor retinaculum	Shaft of metacarpal bone of thumb
Adductor of thumb		
Adductor pollicis	Oblique head: Bases of 2nd–3rd metacarpals; transverse head: Shaft of 3rd metacarpal	Base of proximal phalanx of thumb (medial side)

(Contd.)

Table 9.5: Attachments of small muscles of the hand (Contd.)

Name	Origin	Insertion
Muscle of medial side of palm		
Palmaris brevis	Flexor retinaculum	Skin of palm on medial side
Muscles of hypothenar eminence		
Abductor digiti minimi	Pisiform bone	Base of proximal phalanx of little finger
Flexor digiti minimi	Flexor retinaculum	Base of proximal phalanx of little finger
Opponens digiti minimi	Flexor retinaculum	Medial border of fifth metacarpal bone
Lumbricals		
Lumbricals (4)	1st Lateral side of tendon of 2nd digit	Via extensor expansion into dorsum of
Arise from 4 tendons of flexor	2nd Lateral side of tendon of 3rd digit	bases of distal phalanges
digitorum profundus	3rd Adjacent sides of tendons of 3rd and 4th digits	
	4th Adjacent sides of tendons of 4th and 5th digits	
Palmar interossei—Palmar (4)	1st Medial side of base of 1st metacarpal	Medial side of base of proximal phalanx of thumb or 1st digit
	2nd Medial side of 2nd metacarpal	Via extensor expansion into dorsum of
	3rd Lateral side of 4th metacarpal	bases of distal phalanges of 2nd, 4th
	4th Lateral side of 5th metacarpal	and 5th digits
Dorsal interossei—Dorsal (4)	1st Adjacent sides of 1st and 2nd metacarpals	Via extensor expansion into dorsum of
	2nd Adj. sides of 2nd and 3rd metacarpals	bases of distal phalanges of 2nd, 3rd,
	3rd Adj. sides of 3rd and 4th metacarpals	3rd and 4th digits
	4th Adj. sides of 4th and 5th metacarpals	

Table 9.6: Nerve supply and actions of small muscles of the hand

Muscle	Nerve Supply	Actions
Muscles of Thenar eminence		
Abductor pollicis brevis	Median nerve	Abduction of thumb
Flexor pollicis brevis	Median nerve	Flexes metacarpophalangeal joint of thumb
Opponens pollicis	Median nerve	Pulls thumb medially and forward across palm
Adductor of thumb		
Adductor pollicis	Deep branch of ulnar nerve	Adduction of thumb
Muscle of medial side of palm		
Palmaris brevis	Superficial branch of ulnar nerve	Wrinkles skin to improve grip of palm
Muscles of hypothenar eminences		
Abductor digiti minimi	Deep branch of ulnar nerve	Abducts little finger
Flexor digiti minimi	Deep branch of ulnar nerve	Flexes little finger
Opponens digiti minimi	Deep branch of ulnar nerve	Pulls fifth metacarpal forward as in cupping the palm
Lumbricals		
Lumbricals (4)	First and second, i.e., lateral two by median nerve; third and fourth by deep branch of ulnar nerve	Flex metacarpophalangeal joints, extend interphalangeal joints of 2nd–5th digits
Palmar interossei—Palmar (4)	Deep branch of ulnar nerve	Palmar interossei adduct fingers towards centre of third digit or middle finger
Dorsal interossei—Dorsal (4)	Deep branch of ulnar nerve	Dorsal interossei abduct fingers from centre of third digit; Both palmar and dorsal interossei flex the metacarpophalangeal and extend the interphalangeal joints

Table 9.7: Midpalmar and thenar spaces

Features	Midpalmar space	Thenar space
1. Shape	Triangular	Triangular
2. Situation	Under the inner half of the hollow of the palm	Under the outer half of the hollow of the palm
3. Extent:		
Proximal	Distal margin of the flexor retinaculum	Distal margin of the flexor retinaculum
Distal	Distal palmar crease	Proximal transverse palmar crease
4. Communications:		
Proximal	Forearm space	Forearm space
Distal	Fascial sheaths of the 3rd and 4th lumbricals	Fascial sheath of the first lumbrical
5. Boundaries:		
Anterior	• Flexor tendons of 3rd, 4th and 5th fingers • 2nd, 3rd and 4th lumbricals • Palmar aponeurosis	• Short muscles of thumb • Flexor tendons of the index finger • First lumbrical • Palmar aponeurosis
Posterior	Fascia covering interossei and metacarpals	Transverse head of adductor pollicis
Lateral	Intermediate palmar septum	• Tendon of flexor pollicis longus with radial bursa • Lateral palmar septum
Medial	Medial palmar septum	Intermediate palmar septum
6. Drainage	Incision in either the 3rd or 4th web space	Incision in the first web, posteriorly

structures passing through each compartment, from lateral to the medial side, are listed in Table 9.8 and shown in Fig. 9.2.

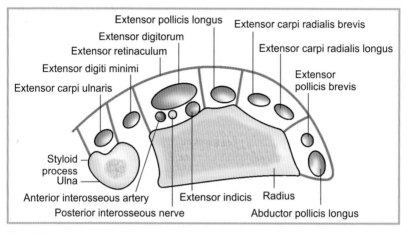

Fig. 9.2: Transverse section passing just above the wrist showing structures passing deep to the extensor retinaculum.

Table 9.8: Structures in various compartments under extensor retinaculum

Compartment	Structure
I	• Abductor pollicis longus • Extensor pollicis brevis
II	• Extensor carpi radialis longus • Extensor carpi radialis brevis
III	• Extensor pollicis longus
IV	• Extensor digitorum • Extensor indicis • Posterior interosseous nerve • Anterior interosseous artery
V	• Extensor digiti minimi
VI	• Extensor carpi ulnaris

SUPERFICIAL MUSCLES

1. Anconeus
2. Brachioradialis
3. Extensor carpi radialis longus
4. Extensor carpi radialis brevis
5. Extensor digitorum
6. Extensor digiti minimi
7. Extensor carpi ulnaris

All the seven muscles cross the elbow joint. Most of them take origin (entirely or in part) from the tip of the lateral epicondyle of the humerus. This is the *common extensor origin* (Tables 9.9 and 9.10).

DEEP MUSCLES

1. Supinator
2. Abductor pollicis longus
3. Extensor pollicis brevis
4. Extensor pollicis longus
5. Extensor indicis

In contrast to the superficial muscles, none of the deep muscles cross the elbow joint. These have been tabulated in Tables 9.11 and 9.12.

CLINICAL ANATOMY

- The radial artery is used for feeling the (arterial) pulse at the wrist. The pulsation can be felt well in this situation because of the presence of the flat radius behind the artery.
- The median nerve controls coarse movements of the hand, as it supplies most of the long muscles of the front of the forearm. It is, therefore, called the *labourer's nerve*.
- When the median nerve is injured above the level of the elbow, as might happen in supracondylar fracture of the humerus, the following features are seen.
  (a) The flexor pollicis longus and lateral half of flexor digitorum profundus are paralysed. The patient is unable to bend the terminal phalanx of the thumb and index finger when the proximal phalanx is held firmly by the clinician (to eliminate the action of the short flexors). Similarly, the terminal phalanx of the middle finger can be tested.
  (b) The forearm is kept in a supine position due to paralysis of the pronators.
  (c) The hand is adducted due to paralysis of the flexor carpi radialis, and flexion at the wrist is weak.
  (d) Flexion at the interphalangeal joints of the index and middle fingers is lost so that the index and to a lesser extent the middle fingers tend to remain straight while making a fist. This is called *pointing index finger* occurs due to paralysis of long flexors of the digit.
  (e) Ape-like thumb deformity is present due to paralysis of the thenar muscles.
  (f) The area of sensory loss corresponds to its distribution in the hand.
  (g) Vasomotor and trophic changes: The skin on lateral three and a half digits is warm, dry and scaly. The nails get cracked easily.

Table 9.9: Attachments of superficial muscles of back of forearm

Name	Origin	Insertion
1. Anconeus	Lateral epicondyle of humerus	Lateral surface of olecranon process of ulna
2. Brachioradialis	Upper 2/3rd of supracondylar ridge of humerus	Base of styloid process of radius
3. Extensor carpi radialis longus	Lower 1/3rd of lateral supracondylar ridge of humerus	Posterior surface of base of second metacarpal bone
4. Extensor carpi radialis brevis	Lateral epicondyle of humerus	Posterior surface of base of third metacarpal bone
5. Extensor digitorum	Lateral epicondyle of humerus	Bases of middle phalanges of the 2nd–5th digits
6. Extensor digiti minimi	Lateral epicondyle of humerus	Extensor expansion of little finger
7. Extensor carpi ulnaris	Lateral epicondyle of humerus	Base of fifth metacarpal bone

Table 9.10: Nerve supply and actions of superficial muscles of back of forearm

Muscle	Nerve Supply	Actions
1. Anconeus	Radial nerve	Extends elbow joint
2. Brachioradialis	Radial nerve	Flexes forearm at elbow joint; rotates forearm to the midprone position from supine or prone positions
3. Extensor carpi radialis longus	Radial nerve	Extends and abducts hand at wrist joint
4. Extensor carpi radialis brevis	Deep branch of radial nerve	Extends and abducts hand at wrist joint
5. Extensor digitorum	Deep branch of radial nerve	Extends fingers of hand
6. Extensor digiti minimi	Deep branch of radial nerve	Extends metacarpophalangeal joint of little finger
7. Extensor carpi ulnaris	Deep branch of radial nerve	Extends and adducts hand at wrist joint

Table 9.11: Attachments of deep muscles of back of forearm

Name	Origin	Insertion
1. Supinator	Lateral epicondyle of humerus, annular ligament of superior radioulnar joint,	Neck and shaft of upper 1/3rd of radius
2. Abductor pollicis longus	Posterior surface of shafts of radius and ulna	Base of first metacarpal bone
3. Extensor pollicis brevis	Posterior surface of shaft of radius	Base of proximal phalanx of thumb
4. Extensor pollicis longus	Posterior surface of shaft of ulna	Base of distal phalanx of thumb
5. Extensor indicis	Posterior surface of shaft of ulna	Extensor expansion of index finger

Table 9.12: Nerve supply and actions of deep muscles of back of forearm

Muscle	Nerve Supply	Actions
1. Supinator	Deep branch of radial nerve	Supination of forearm when elbow is extended
2. Abductor pollicis longus	Deep branch of radial nerve	Abducts and extends thumb
3. Extensor pollicis brevis	Deep branch of radial nerve	Extends metacarpophalangeal joint of thumb
4. Extensor pollicis longus	Deep branch of radial nerve	Extends distal phalanx of thumb
5. Extensor indicis	Deep branch of radial nerve	Extends metacarpophalangeal joint of index finger

- *Median nerve injury at the wrist:* This is a common occurrence and is characterised by the following signs.
  - (a) The median nerve controls coarse movements of the hand and is the *eye of the hand* as it is sensory to most of the hand. In all injuries of this nerve, at whatever level, the patient is unable to pick up a pin with the thumb and index finger. In fact, inability to oppose the thumb is the chief disability of median nerve lesions at the wrist.
  - (b) *Ape-like hand:* Paralysis of the short muscles of the thumb, and the unopposed action of the extensor pollicis longus produces an ape-like hand. The thenar eminence is wasted and flattened. The thumb is adducted and laterally rotated so that the first metacarpal lies in the same plane as the other metacarpals..
  - (c) *Pen test for abductor pollicis brevis:* Lay the hand flat on a table with the palm directed upwards. The patient is unable to touch with his thumb a pen held in front of the palm.
  - (d) *Test for opponens pollicis:* Request the patient to touch the proximal phalanx of 2nd to 5th digits with the tip of thumb.
  - (e) Paralysis of the first and second lumbricals makes the index and middle fingers lag behind in slowly making a fist leading to their *partial clawing*. The sensory loss, vasomotor and trophic changes are similar to that seen in lesions of the nerve at the elbow.
  - (f) Sensory loss corresponds to distribution of the median nerve in the hand.

  As already mentioned, median nerve lesions are more disabling than ulnar nerve lesions. This is largely due to the inability to oppose the thumb, so that the gripping action of the hand is totally lost.
- *Carpal tunnel syndrome:* Involvement of the median nerve in carpal tunnel has become a very common entity (Fig. 9.1).
- This syndrome consists of motor, sensory, vasomotor and trophic symptoms in the hand caused by compression of the median nerve in the carpal tunnel. Examination reveals wasting of thenar eminence (ape-like hand), hypoaesthesia to light touch on the palmar aspect of lateral 3½ digits. However, the skin over the thenar eminence is not affected as the branch of median nerve supplying it arises in the forearm.
- *Motor changes:* Ape-like thumb deformity, loss of opposition of thumb, index and middle fingers lag behind while making the fist due to paralysis of 1st and 2nd lumbrical muscles and their partial clawing.
- *Sensory changes:* Loss of sensations on lateral 3½ digits including the nail beds and distal phalanges on dorsum of hand.
- *Vasomotor changes:* The skin areas with sensory loss is warmer due to arteriolar dilatation. It is also drier due to absence of sweating because of loss of sympathetic supply.

- *Trophic changes:* Long-standing cases of paralysis lead to dry and scaly skin. The nails crack easily with atrophy of the pulp of fingers.
- It occurs both in males and in females between the ages of 25 and 70. They complain of intermittent attacks of pain in the distribution of the median nerve on one or both sides. The attacks frequently occur at night. Pain may be referred proximally to the forearm and arm. It is more common because of excessive working on the computer. Phalen's test is attempted for carpal tunnel syndrome.
- ***Dupuytren's contracture:*** This condition is due to inflammation involving the ulnar side of the palmar aponeurosis. There is thickening and contraction of the aponeurosis. As a result, the proximal phalanx and later the middle phalanx become flexed and cannot be straightened. The terminal phalanx remains unaffected. The ring finger is most commonly involved.
- Paralysis of the intrinsic muscles of the hand produces *claw-hand* in which there is hyperextension at the metacarpophalangeal joints, and flexion at the interphalangeal joints. (The effect is opposite to the action of the lumbricals and interossei.)
- Testing the muscles
  (a) The dorsal interossei are tested by asking the subject to spread out the fingers against resistance.
  (b) The palmar interossei and adductor pollicis are tested by placing a piece of paper between the fingers, between thumb and index finger, and seeing how firmly it can be held.
  (c) The lumbricals and interossei are tested by asking the subject to flex the fingers at the metacarpophalangeal joints against resistance.
- The ulnar nerve is also known as the *musician's nerve* because it controls fine movements of the fingers.
- The ulnar nerve is commonly injured at the elbow, behind the medial epicondyle or distal to elbow as it passes between two heads of flexor carpi ulnaris (cubital tunnel) or at the wrist in front of the flexor retinaculum.
  When the nerve is injured at the elbow, the flexor carpi ulnaris and the medial half of the flexor digitorum profundus are paralysed.
- Due to this paralysis the medial border of the forearm becomes flattened. An attempt to produce flexion at the wrist result in abduction of the hand. The tendon of the flexor carpi ulnaris does not tighten on making a fist. Flexion of the terminal phalanges of the ring and little fingers is lost.
- The ulnar nerve controls fine movements of the fingers through its extensive motor distribution to the short muscles of the hand.
- An ulnar nerve lesion at the wrist produces *ulnar claw-hand.*

- *Ulnar claw-hand* is characterised by the following signs.
  (a) Hyperextension at the metacarpophalangeal joints and flexion at the interphalangeal joints, involving the ring and little fingers—more than the index and middle fingers. The little finger is held in extension by extensor muscles. The intermetacarpal spaces are hollowed out due to wasting of the interosseous muscles. Claw-hand deformity is more obvious in wrist lesions as the profundus muscle is spared: This causes marked flexion of the terminal phalanges (action of paradox).
  (b) *Sensory loss* is confined to the medial one-third of the palm and the medial one and a half fingers including their nail beds.
  (c) *Vasomotor changes:* The skin areas with sensory loss is warmer due to arteriolar dilatation; it is also drier due to absence of sweating because of loss of sympathetic supply.
  (d) *Trophic changes:* Long-standing cases of paralysis lead to dry and scaly skin. The nails crack easily with atrophy of the pulp of fingers.
  (e) The patient is unable to spread out the fingers due to paralysis of the dorsal interossei. The power of adduction of the thumb, and flexion of the ring and little fingers are lost. It should be noted that median nerve lesions are more disabling. In contrast, ulnar nerve lesions leave a relatively efficient hand.
- Ulnar nerve injury at the wrist can be tested by *Froment's sign*, or the book test which tests the adductor pollicis muscle. When the patient is asked to grasp a book firmly between the thumb and other fingers of both the hands, the terminal phalanx of the thumb on the paralysed side becomes flexed at the interphalangeal joint (by the flexor pollicis longus which is supplied by the median nerve).
- If both median and ulnar nerves are paralysed, the result is complete claw-hand.

Joints of Upper Limb

SHOULDER GIRDLE

Sternoclavicular Joint

The sternoclavicular joint is a synovial joint. It is a complex joint as its cavity is subdivided into two compartments: medial and lateral by an intra-articular disc (Fig. 10.1).

The *capsular ligament* is attached laterally to the margins of the clavicular articular surface; and medially to the margins of the articular areas on the sternum and on the first costal cartilage. However, the main bond of union at this joint is the *articular disc.*

There are two other ligaments associated with this joint. The *interclavicular* ligament and the *costoclavicular ligament.*

Acromioclavicular Joint

The acromioclavicular joint is a plane synovial joint. It is formed by articulation of small facets present:
  (i) At the lateral end of the clavicle.
 (ii) On the medial margin of the acromion process of the scapula.

The bones are held together by a fibrous capsule and by the articular disc.

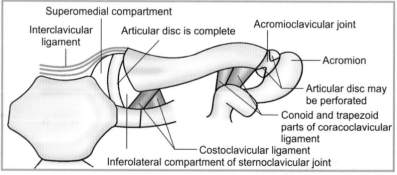

Fig. 10.1: The sternoclavicular and acromioclavicular joints.

CORACOCLAVICULAR LIGAMENT

The ligament consists of two parts—conoid and trapezoid. The trapezoid part is attached, below to the upper surface of the coracoid process; and above to the trapezoid line on the inferior surface of the lateral one-third part of the clavicle. The conoid part is attached, below to the root of the coracoid process just lateral to the scapular notch. It is attached above to the inferior surface of the clavicle on the conoid tubercle.

Movements of the Shoulder Girdle

Movements at the two joints of the girdle are always associated with the movements of the scapula (Fig. 10.2).

1. *Elevation* of the scapula (as in shrugging the shoulders). The movement is brought about by the upper fibres of the trapezius and by the levator scapulae.
2. *Depression* of the scapula (drooping of the shoulder). It is brought about by gravity, and actively by the lower fibres of the serratus anterior and by the pectoralis minor.
3. *Protraction* of the scapula (as in pushing and punching movements). It is brought about by the serratus anterior.

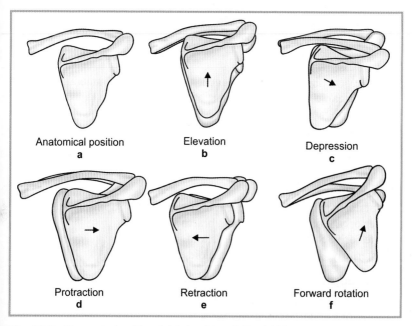

Fig. 10.2: Movements of the right shoulder girdle. (a) The anatomical position. The underlying scapulae in (b) to (f) are also in anatomical position. The overlying scapulae with arrows show their respective movement.

4. *Retraction* of the scapula (squaring the shoulders) is brought about by the rhomboideus and by the middle fibres of the trapezius.
5. *Forward rotation* of the scapula round the chest wall takes place during overhead abduction of the arm. The scapula rotates around the coracoclavicular ligament. The movement is brought about by the upper fibres of the trapezius and the lower fibres of the serratus anterior.
6. *Backward rotation* of the scapula occurs under the influence of gravity, although it can be brought about actively by the levator scapulae and the rhomboideus.

SHOULDER JOINT

The shoulder joint is a synovial joint of the ball and socket variety.

Articular Surface

Structurally, it is a weak joint because the glenoid cavity is too small and shallow to hold the head of the humerus in place. Stability of the joint is maintained by the following factors.
1. The coracoacromial arch or secondary socket for the head of the humerus.
2. The musculotendinous cuff of the shoulder formed by subscapularis supraspinatus, infraspinatus and teres minor muscles.
3. The glenoidal labrum helps in deepening the glenoid fossa.

Ligaments

- As the articular capsule is opened, the three glenohumeral ligaments are noticeable on the anterior part of the capsule.
- Capsular ligament
- Coracohumeral ligament
- Transverse humeral ligament
- Glenoidal labrum

Relations

- Superiorly (Fig. 10.3): Coracoacromial arch and supraspinatus
- Inferiorly: Long head of triceps brachii
- Anteriorly: Subscapularis and deltoid
- Posteriorly: Infraspinatus and deltoid

Blood Supply

- Anterior circumflex humeral vessels
- Posterior circumflex humeral vessels
- Suprascapular vessels
- Subscapular vessels

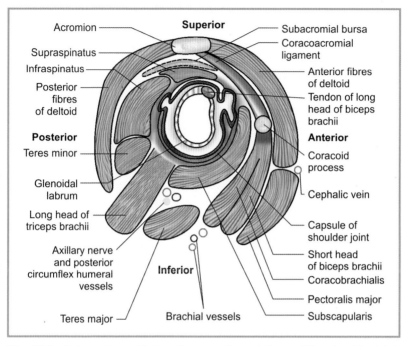

Fig. 10.3: Schematic sagittal section showing relations of the shoulder joint.

Nerve Supply

- Axillary nerve
- Musculocutaneous nerve
- Suprascapular nerve

Movements at Shoulder Joint

Table 10.1.

ELBOW JOINT

Upper

The capitulum and trochlea of the humerus.

Lower

(i) Upper surface of the head of radius articulates with the capitulum.

(ii) Trochlear notch of the ulna articulates with the trochlea of the humerus (Fig. 10.4).

The elbow joint is continuous with the superior radioulnar joint. The humeroradial, the humeroulnar and the superior radioulnar joints are together known as cubital articulations.

Table 10.1: Muscles bringing about movements at the shoulder joint

Movements	Main muscles	Accessory muscles
1. Flexion	• Clavicular head of the pectoralis major • Anterior fibres of deltoid	• Coracobrachialis • Short head of biceps brachii
2. Extension	• Posterior fibres of deltoid • Latissimus dorsi	• Teres major • Long head of triceps brachii • Sternocostal head of the pectoralis major
3. Adduction	• Pectoralis major • Latissimus dorsi • Short head of biceps brachii • Long head of triceps brachii	• Teres major • Coracobrachialis
4. Abduction	• Supraspinatus 0°–15° controversial • Deltoid 0°–90° • Serratus anterior 90°–180° • Upper and lower fibres of trapezius 90°–180°	—
5. Medial rotation	• Pectoralis major • Anterior fibres of deltoid • Latissimus dorsi • Teres major	• Subscapularis
6. Lateral rotation	• Posterior fibres of deltoid • Infraspinatus • Teres minor	—

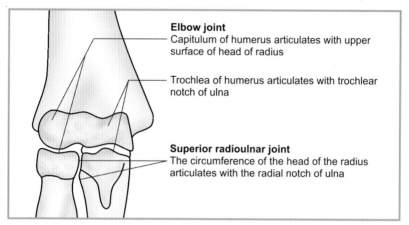

Elbow joint
Capitulum of humerus articulates with upper surface of head of radius

Trochlea of humerus articulates with trochlear notch of ulna

Superior radioulnar joint
The circumference of the head of the radius articulates with the radial notch of ulna

Fig. 10.4: The cubital articulations, including the elbow and superior radioulnar joints.

Ligaments

1. Capsular ligament
2. Anterior ligament
3. Posterior ligament
4. Ulnar collateral ligament
5. Radial collateral or lateral ligament

Movements

1. Flexion is brought about by
   (i) Brachialis
   (ii) Biceps brachii
   (iii) Brachioradialis.
2. Extension is produced by
   (i) Triceps brachii
   (ii) Anconeus

RADIOULNAR JOINTS

The radius and the ulna are joined to each other at the superior and inferior radioulnar joints. These are described in Table 10.2. The radius and ulna are also connected by the interosseous membrane which constitutes middle radioulnar joint (Fig. 10.5).

Interosseous Membrane

The interosseous membrane connects the shafts of the radius and ulna. It is attached to the interosseous borders of these bones. The fibres of the membrane run downwards and medially from the radius to ulna.

Table 10.2: Radioulnar joints (Fig. 10.5)

Features	Superior radioulnar joint	Inferior radioulnar joint
Type	Pivot type of synovial joint	Pivot type of synovial joint
Articular surfaces	• Circumference of head of radius • Osseofibrous ring, formed by the radial notch of the ulna and the annular ligament	• Head of ulna • Ulnar notch of radius
Ligaments	• The annular ligament. It forms four-fifths of the ring within which the head of the radius rotates. It is attached to the margins of the radial notch of the ulna, and is continuous with the capsule of the elbow joint above. • The quadrate ligament, extends from the neck of the radius to the lower margin of the radial notch of the ulna	• The capsule surrounds the joint. The weak upper part is evaginated by the synovial membrane to form a recess (recessus sacciformis) in front of the interosseous membrane • The apex of articular disc is attached to the base of the styloid process of the ulna, and the base to the lower margin of the ulnar notch of the radius
Blood supply	Anastomoses around the lateral side of the elbow joint	Anterior and posterior interosseous arteries
Nerve supply	Musculocutaneous, median, and radial nerves	Anterior and posterior interosseous nerves
Movements	Supination and pronation	Supination and pronation

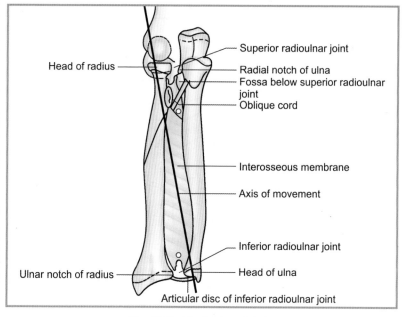

Fig. 10.5: Radioulnar joints.

WRIST (RADIOCARPAL) JOINT

Wrist joint is a synovial joint of the ellipsoid variety between lower end of radius and three lateral bones of proximal row of carpus.

Articular Surfaces

Upper

1. Inferior surface of the lower end of the radius.
2. Articular disc of the inferior radioulnar joint (Fig. 10.6).

Lower

1 Scaphoid
2. Lunate
3. Triquetral (only during adduction of wrist)

Ligaments

1. Articular capsule
2. Palmar radiocarpal ligament
3. Dorsal radiocarpal ligament
4. Radial collateral ligament
5. Ulnar collateral ligament

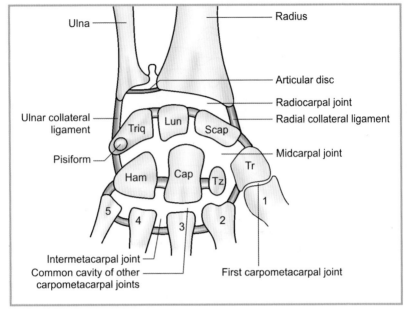

Fig. 10.6: Joints in the region of the wrist.

Movements

1. *Flexion:* It takes place more at the midcarpal than at the wrist joint. The main flexors are:
   (i) Flexor carpi radialis.
   (ii) Flexor carpi ulnaris.

2. *Extension*
   (i) Extensor carpi radialis longus.
   (ii) Extensor carpi radialis brevis.
   (iii) Extensor carpi ulnaris.

3. *Abduction:* It occurs mainly at the midcarpal joint. The main abductors are:
   (i) Flexor carpi radialis.
   (ii) Extensor carpi radialis longus and extensor carpi radialis brevis.
   (iii) Abductor pollicis longus and extensor pollicis brevis.

4. *Adduction:* It occurs mainly at the wrist joint. The main adductors are:
   (i) Flexor carpi ulnaris.
   (ii) Extensor carpi ulnaris.

5. *Circumduction:* The range of flexion is more than that of extension. Similarly the range of adduction is greater than abduction (due to the shorter styloid process of ulna).

JOINTS OF HAND

INTERCARPAL, CARPOMETACARPAL AND INTERMETACARPAL JOINTS

There are three joint cavities among the intercarpal, carpometacarpal and intermetacarpal joints, which are:
1. Pisotriquetral
2. First carpometacarpal
3. A common cavity for the rest of the joints; the common cavity may be described as the *midcarpal* (transverse intercarpal) joint between the proximal and distal rows of the carpus

FIRST CARPOMETACARPAL JOINT

Saddle variety of synovial joint (because the articular surfaces are concavoconvex).

Articular Surfaces

 (i) The distal surface of the trapezium
(ii) The proximal surface of the base of the first metacarpal bone.

Ligaments

1. Capsular ligament
2. Lateral ligament
3. Anterior ligament
4. Posterior ligament

Movements

Flexion and extension of the thumb take place in the plane of the palm, and abduction and adduction at right angles to the plane of the palm. In opposition, the thumb crosses the palm and touches other fingers. Flexion is associated with medial rotation, and extension with lateral rotation at the joint. Circumduction is a combination of different movements mentioned. The following muscles bring about the movements.

1. Flexion	• Flexor pollicis brevis
	• Opponens pollicis
2. Extension	• Extensor pollicis brevis
	• Extensor pollicis longus
3. Abduction	• Abductor pollicis brevis
	• Abductor pollicis longus
4. Adduction	• Adductor pollicis
5. Opposition	• Opponens pollicis
	• Flexor pollicis brevis

The adductor pollicis and the flexor pollicis longus exert pressure on the opposed fingers.

METACARPOPHALANGEAL JOINTS

Metacarpophalangeal joints are synovial joints of the ellipsoid variety.

Ligaments

Each joint has the following ligaments
1. Capsular ligament
2. Palmar ligament
3. Medial and lateral collateral ligaments

Movements at first joint and muscles producing them
1. *Flexion:* Flexor pollicis longus and flexor pollicis brevis
2. *Extension:* Extensor pollicis longus and extensor pollicis brevis
3. *Abduction:* Abductor pollicis brevis
4. *Adduction:* Adductor pollicis

Movements at second to fifth joints and muscles producing them
1. *Flexion:* Interossei and lumbricals
2. *Extension:* Extensors of the fingers
3. *Abduction:* Dorsal interossei
4. *Adduction:* Palmar interossei
5. *Circumduction:* Above muscles in sequence

INTERPHALANGEAL JOINTS (PROXIMAL AND DISTAL)

Hinge variety of synovial joints

Ligaments

Similar to the metacarpophalangeal joints, that is one palmar fibrocartilaginous ligament and two collateral bands running downwards and forwards.

Movements at Interphalangeal Joint of Thumb

1. *Flexion:* Flexor pollicis longus
2. *Extension:* Extensor pollicis longus

Movements at Second to Fifth Digits

1. *Flexion*: Flexor digitorum superficialis at the proximal interphalangeal joint, and the flexor digitorum profundus at the distal joint.
2. *Extension:* Interossei and lumbricals

Segmental Innervation of Movements of Upper Limb

Figure 10.7 shows the segments of the spinal cord responsible for movements of the various joints of the upper limb.

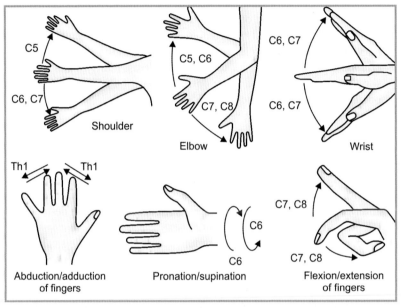

Fig. 10.7: Segmental innervation of movements of the upper limb.

CLINICAL ANATOMY

- The clavicle may be dislocated at either of its ends. At the medial end, it is usually dislocated forwards. Backward dislocation is rare as it is prevented by the costoclavicular ligament.
- The main bond of union between the clavicle and the manubrium is the articular disc. Apart from its attachment to the joint capsule the disc is also attached above to the medial end of the clavicle, and below to the manubrium. This prevents the sternal end of the clavicle from tilting upwards when the weight of the arm depresses the acromial end (Fig. 10.1).
- The clavicle dislocates upwards at the acromioclavicular joint, because the clavicle overrides the acromion.
- The weight of the limb is transmitted from the scapula to the clavicle through the coracoclavicular ligament, and from the clavicle to the sternum through the sternoclavicular joint. Some of the weight also passes to the first rib by the costoclavicular ligament. The clavicle usually fractures between these two ligaments (Fig. 10.1).

- *Dislocation:* The shoulder joint is more prone to dislocation than any other joint. This is due to laxity of the capsule and the disproportionate area of the articular surfaces. Dislocation usually occurs when the arm is abducted. In this position, the head of the humerus presses against the lower unsupported part of the capsular ligament. Thus almost always the dislocation is primarily subglenoid. Dislocation endangers the axillary nerve which is closely related to the lower part of the joint capsule.
- *Optimum position:* In order to avoid ankylosis, many diseases of the shoulder joint are treated in an optimum position of the joint. In this position, the arm is abducted by 45–90 degrees.
- *Shoulder tip pain:* Irritation of the peritoneum underlying diaphragm from any surrounding pathology causes referred pain in the shoulder. This is so because the phrenic nerve and the supraclavicular nerves (supplying the skin over the shoulder) both arise from spinal segment C4.
- The shoulder joint is most commonly approached (surgically) from the front. However, for aspiration the needle may be introduced either anteriorly through the deltopectoral triangle (closer to the deltoid), or laterally just below the acromion.
- *Frozen shoulder:* This is a common occurrence. Pathologically, the two layers of the synovial membrane become adherent to each other. Clinically, the patient (usually 40–60 years of age) complains of progressively increasing pain in the shoulder, stiffness in the joint and restriction of some movements. The surrounding muscles show disuse atrophy. The disease is self-limiting and the patient may recover spontaneously in about two years.
- Shoulder joint disease can be excluded if the patient can raise both his arms above the head and bring the two palms together. Deltoid muscle and axillary nerve are likely to be intact.
- *Distension* of the elbow joint by an effusion occurs posteriorly because here the capsule is weak and the covering deep fascia is thin. Aspiration is done posteriorly on any side of the olecranon.
- *Dislocation* of the elbow is usually posterior, and is often associated with fracture of the coronoid process. The triangular relationship between the olecranon and the two humeral epicondyles is lost.
- *Subluxation* of the head of the radius (pulled elbow) occurs in children when the forearm is suddenly pulled in pronation. The head of the radius slips out from the annular ligament.
- *Tennis elbow:* Occurs in tennis players. Abrupt pronation with fully extended elbow may lead to pain and tenderness over the lateral epicondyle. This is possibly due to:
  (a) Sprain of radial collateral ligament.
  (b) Tearing of fibres of the extensor carpi radialis brevis.

- *Student's* (or *Miner's elbow*) is characterised by effusion into the bursa over the subcutaneous posterior surface of the olecranon process. Students during lectures support their head (for sleeping) with their hands with flexed elbows. The bursa on the olecranon process gets inflamed.
- *Golfer's elbow* is the microtrauma of medial epicondyle of humerus, occurs, commonly in golf players.
- If carrying angle (normal is 13°) is more, the condition is *cubitus valgus*, ulnar nerve may get stretched leading to weakness of intrinsic muscles of hand. If the angle is less it is called as *cubitus varus*.
- *Supination and pronation:* During supination the radius and ulna are parallel to each other. During pronation radius crosses over the ulna. In synostosis (fusion) of upper end of radius and ulna, pronation is not possible.
- The wrist joint and interphalangeal joints are commonly involved in *rheumatoid arthritis*.
- The back of the wrist is the common site for a *ganglion*. It is a cystic swelling resulting from mucoid degeneration of synovial sheaths around the tendons.
- The wrist joint can be aspirated from the posterior surface between the tendons of the extensor pollicis longus and the extensor digitorum.
- The joint is immobilised in optimum position of 30 degrees dorsiflexion (extension).

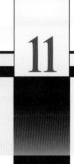

Surface Marking

ARTERIES

Axillary Artery

Hold the arm at right angle to the trunk with the palm directed upwards. The artery is then marked as a straight line by joining the following two points.

  (i) Midpoint of the clavicle

 (ii) The second point at the lower limit of the lateral wall of axilla where the arterial pulsations can be felt in living person.

At its termination, the axillary artery, along with the accompanying nerves, forms a prominence which lies behind another projection caused by the biceps and coracobrachialis.

Brachial Artery

Brachial artery is marked by joining the following two points.

  (i) A point at the lower limit of the lateral wall of the axilla. Here the axillary artery ends and the brachial artery begins.

 (ii) The second point, at the level of the neck of the radius medial to the tendons of the biceps brachii.

Thus the artery begins on the medial side of the upper part of the arm, and runs downwards and slightly laterally to end in front of the elbow. At its termination it bifurcates into the radial and ulnar arteries.

Superficial Palmar Arch

Superficial palmar arch is formed by the direct continuation of the ulnar artery, and is marked as a curved line by joining the following points.

  (i) A point just lateral and distal to the pisiform bone

 (ii) The second point on the hook of the hamate bone

(iii) The third point on the distal border of the thenar eminence in line with the cleft between the index and middle fingers.

The convexity of the arch is directed towards the fingers, and its most distal point is situated at the level of the distal border of the fully extended thumb.

Deep Palmar Arch

Deep palmar arch is formed as the direct continuation of the radial artery. It has a slight convexity towards the fingers. It is marked by a more or less horizontal line, 4 cm long, just distal to the hook of the hamate bone.

The deep palmar arch lies 1.2 cm proximal to the superficial palmar arch across the metacarpals, immediately distal to their bases. The deep branch of ulnar nerve lies in its concavity.

NERVES

Axillary Nerve with its Divisions

Axillary nerve with its divisions is marked as a horizontal line on the deltoid muscle, 2 cm above the midpoint between the tip of the acromion process and the insertion of the deltoid.

Intramuscular injections in the deltoid are given in the middle part of the muscle to avoid injury to the axillary nerve and its accompanying vessels.

RETINACULA

Flexor Retinaculum

Flexor retinaculum is marked by joining the following four points.
  (i) Pisiform bone
 (ii) Tubercle of the scaphoid bone
(iii) Hook of the hamate bone
 (iv) Crest of the trapezium

The upper border is obtained by joining the first and second points, and the lower border by joining the third and fourth points. The upper border is concave upwards, and the lower border is concave downwards.

Extensor Retinaculum

Extensor retinaculum is an oblique band directed downwards and medially, and is about 2 cm broad (vertically). Laterally, it is attached to the lower salient part of the anterior border of the radius, and medially to the medial side of the carpus (pisiform and triquetral bones) and to the styloid process of the ulna.

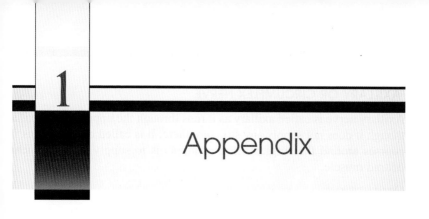

Appendix

Since **nerves** are the very important and precious component of our body, this appendix deals with the nerves of the upper limb. Most of the nerves course through different regions of the upper limb and have been described in parts in the respective regions. In this appendix, the course of the entire nerve from origin to its termination including the branches and clinical aspects has been described briefly. **Arteries** of upper limb have been tabulated in Table A1.5. Important **clinical terms** related to upper limb have been defined.

MUSCULOCUTANEOUS NERVE

Musculocutaneous nerve is so named as it supplies muscles of front of arm and skin of lateral side of forearm.

Root Value
Ventral rami of C5, C6 and C7 segments of spinal cord.

Course
Musculocutaneous nerve is a branch of the lateral cord of brachial plexus, lies lateral to axillary and upper part of brachial artery. It supplies coracobrachialis, pierces the muscle to lie in the intermuscular septum between biceps brachii and brachialis muscles, both of which are supplied by this nerve. At the crease of elbow it becomes cutaneous by piercing the deep fascia. The nerve is called the lateral cutaneous nerve of forearm which supplies skin of lateral side of forearm both on the front and on the back.

Branches

Muscular	Coracobrachialis, long head of biceps brachii, short head of biceps brachii, and brachialis.
Cutaneous	Lateral side of forearm (both on the front and on the back.)
Articular	Elbow joint

This nerve rarely gets injured.

AXILLARY OR CIRCUMFLEX NERVE

Axillary nerve is called axillary as it runs through the upper part of axilla though it does not supply any structure there. It is called circumflex as it courses around the surgical neck of humerus to supply the prominent deltoid muscle.

Root Value

Ventral rami of C5, C6 segments of spinal cord.

Course

Axillary or circumflex nerve is the smaller terminal branch of posterior cord. It passes backwards through the quadrangular space (bounded by subscapularis above, teres major below, long head of triceps brachii medially and surgical neck of humerus laterally). Here it lies below the capsule of the shoulder joint. As it is about to pass behind the surgical neck of humerus it divides into an anterior and posterior divisions.

Branches

The branches of axillary nerve are presented in Table A1.1.

RADIAL NERVE

Radial nerve is the thickest branch of brachial plexus.

Root Value

Ventral rami of C5–C8, T1 segments of spinal cord.

Course

Axilla

Radial nerve lies against the muscles forming the posterior wall of axilla, i.e. subscapularis, teres major and latissimus dorsi. It then lies in the lower triangular space between teres major, long head of triceps brachii and shaft of humerus. It gives two muscular and one cutaneous branch in the axilla.

Radial sulcus

Radial nerve enters through the lower triangular space into the radial sulcus, where it lies between the long and medial heads of triceps brachii along with profunda brachii vessels. Long and lateral heads form the roof of the radial sulcus. It leaves the sulcus by piercing the lateral intermuscular septum. In the sulcus, it gives three muscular and two cutaneous branches.

Front of arm

Radial nerve enters the lower anterolateral part of arm and lies between brachialis on the medial side and brachioradialis with extensor carpi radialis longus on the lateral side. It supplies the latter two muscles and also brachialis (lateral part). The nerve descends deep in this interval to reach the cubital fossa, where it ends by dividing into its two terminal branches—the superficial and deep or posterior interosseous branches.

Posterior interosseous branch

Lies in the lateral part of cubital fossa, where it supplies extensor carpi radialis brevis and supinator muscles. Then it enters into the back of forearm by passing through supinator muscle. There the nerve supplies abductor pollicis longus, extensor pollicis brevis, extensor pollicis longus, extensor digitorum, extensor indicis, extensor digiti minimi and extensor carpi ulnaris. It ends in a pseudoganglion, branches of which supply the wrist joint.

Superficial branch

Superficial branch is given off in the cubital fossa and runs on the lateral side of forearm accompanied by radial artery in the upper two-thirds of forearm. Then it curves posteriorly to descend till the anatomical snuff box. It gives branches to supply the skin of lateral half of dorsum of hand and lateral two and a half digits till distal interphalangeal joints.

Branches of Radial Nerve

The branches of radial nerve are presented in Table A1.2.

MEDIAN NERVE

Median nerve is called median as it runs in the median plane of the forearm.

Root Value

Ventral rami of C5–C8, T1 segments of spinal cord.

Course

Axilla

Median nerve is formed by two roots, lateral root from lateral cord and medial root from medial cord of brachial plexus. Medial root crosses the axillary artery to join the lateral root. The median nerve runs on the lateral side of axillary artery.

Arm

Median nerve continues to run on the lateral side of brachial artery till the middle of arm, where it crosses in front of the artery, passes anterior to elbow joint into the forearm.

Forearm

Median nerve passes through cubital fossa lying medial to the brachial artery. It leaves the fossa between two heads of pronator teres where it gives anterior interosseous branch. Then it lies deep to fibrous arch of flexor digitorum superficialis. Adheres to deep surface of flexor digitorum superficialis, leaves the muscle, along its lateral border. Lastly it is placed deep and lateral to palmaris longus to enter palm under the flexor retinaculum. It gives number of branches in cubital fossa and forearm.

Palm
Median nerve lies medial to the muscles of thenar eminence, which it supplies. It also gives cutaneous branches to lateral three and a half digits and their nail beds including skin of distal phalanges on their dorsal aspect.

Branches of median nerve
The branches of median nerve are presented in Table A1.3.

ULNAR NERVE

Ulnar nerve is named so as it runs along the medial or ulnar side of the upper limb.

Root value: Ventral rami of C8 and T1. It also gets fibres of C7 from the lateral root of median nerve.

Course

Axilla
Ulnar nerve lies in the axilla between the axillary vein and axillary artery on a deeper plane. Lies medial to brachial artery. Runs downwards with the brachial artery in its proximal part. At the middle of arm it pierces the medial intermuscular septum to lie on its back and descends on the back of medial epicondyle of humerus where it can be palpated. Palpation causes tingling sensations. That is why humerus is called "funny bone".

Forearm
Ulnar nerve enters the forearm by passing between two heads of flexor carpi ulnaris. There it lies on medial part of flexor digitorum profundus. It is accompanied by the ulnar artery in lower two-thirds of forearm. It gives two muscular and two cutaneous branches (Table A1.4). Finally it lies on the medial part of flexor retinaculum to enter palm. At the distal border of retinaculum the nerve divides into its superficial and deep branches.

Palm
Superficial branch supplies palmaris brevis and digital branches to medial one and a half digits. Deep branch supplies most of the intrinsic muscles of the hand. At first it supplies three muscles of hypothenar eminence; running in the concavity of deep palmar arch it gives branches to 4th and 3rd lumbricals from deep aspect, 4,3,2,1 dorsal interossei and 4,3,2,1 palmar interossei to end in adductor pollicis. Since it supplies intrinsic

Table A1.1: Branches of axillary nerve

	Trunk	Anterior division	Posterior division
Muscular	—	Deltoid (most part)	Deltoid (posterior part) and teres minor. The nerve to teres minor is characterised by the presence of a pseudoganglion
Cutaneous	—	—	Upper lateral cutaneous nerve of arm
Articular and vascular	Shoulder joint	—	To posterior circumflex humeral artery

Table A1.2: Branches of radial nerve

	Axilla	Radial sulcus	Lateral side of arm
Muscular	Long head of triceps brachii Medial head of triceps brachii	Lateral head of triceps brachii Medial head of triceps brachii Anconeus	Brachioradialis Extensor carpi radialis longus Lateral part of brachialis proprioceptive
Cutaneous	Posterior cutaneous nerve	Posterior cutaneous nerve of forearm Lower lateral cutaneous nerve of arm	—
Vascular	—	To profunda brachii artery	—
Terminal	—	—	Superficial and deep or posterior interosseous branches

Table A1.3: Branches of median nerve

	Axilla and arm	Cubital fossa	Forearm	Palm
Muscular	Pronator teres in lower part of arm	Flexor carpi radialis, flexor digitorum superficialis, palmaris longus	Anterior interosseous which supplies: lateral half of flexor digitorum profundus, pronator quadratus, and flexor pollicis longus	Recurrent branch for abductor pollicis brevis, flexor pollicis brevis, opponens pollicis, 1st lumbrical and 2nd lumbrical from the digital nerves
Cutaneous	—	—	Palmar cutaneous branch for lateral two-thirds of palm	• Two digital branches to lateral and medial sides of thumb, • One to lateral side of index finger • Two to adjacent sides of index and middle fingers • Two to adjacent sides middle and ring fingers. These branches also supply dorsal aspects of distal phalanges of lateral three and a half digits
Articular and vascular	Brachial artery	Elbow joint	—	Gives vascular and articular branches to joints of hand

muscles of hand responsible for finer movements, this nerve is called 'musician's nerve'.

Branches

The branches of ulnar nerve are presented in Table A1.4.

Table A1.4: Branches of ulnar nerve

	Forearm	Hand
Muscular	Medial half of flexor digitorum profundus, flexor carpi ulnaris	Superficial branch; palmaris brevis. Deep branch-Hypothenar eminence muscles, medial two lumbricals, 4–1 dorsal and palmar interossei and adductor pollicis
Cutaneous/ Digital	Dorsal cutaneous branch for medial half of dorsum of hand. Palmar cutaneous branch for medial one-third of palm. Digital branches to medial one and a half fingers, nail beds and dorsal distal phalanges	—
Vascular/ Articular	Also supplies digital vessels and joints of medial side of hand	—

CLINICAL ANATOMY

Shoulder joint is mostly dislocated inferiorly: The shoulder joint is surrounded by short muscles on all aspects except inferiorly. Since the joint is quite mobile it dislocates at the unprotected site, i.e. inferiorly.

Students' elbow: Inflammation of the bursa over the insertion of triceps brachii is called student's elbow. It is common in students as they use the flexed elbow to support the head while attempting hard to listen to the lectures in between their 'naps'.

Tennis elbow: Lateral epicondylitis occurs in players of lawn tennis or table tennis. The extensor muscles of forearm are used to hit the ball sharply, causing repeated *microtrauma* to the lateral epicondyle and its subsequent inflammation.

Pulled elbow: While pulling the children by their hands (getting them off the bus) the head of radius may slip out of the annular ligament. Annular ligament is not tight in children as in adults, so the head of radius slips out.

Table A1.5: Arteries of upper limb

Artery	Origin, course and termination	Area of distribution
AXILLARY	Starts at the outer border of first rib as continuation of subclavian artery, runs through axilla and continues as brachial artery at the lower border of teres major muscle.	Supplies all walls of axilla, pectoral region including mammary gland.
Superior thoracic	From 1st part of axillary artery	Supplies upper part of thoracic wall and the pectoral muscles
Thoracoacromial	From 2nd part of axillary artery, pierces clavipectoral fascia and divides into branches: acromial, pectoral, clavicular and deltoid	Supplies pectoral and deltoid muscles
Lateral thoracic	From 2nd part of axillary artery runs along inferolateral border of pectoralis minor	Supplies the muscles of thoracic wall including the mammary gland
Anterior circumflex humeral	From third part of axillary artery, runs on the anterior aspect of intertubercular sulcus and anastomoses with large posterior circumflex humeral artery	Supplies the neighbouring shoulder joint and the muscles
Posterior circumflex humeral	From third part of axillary artery, lies along the surgical neck of humerus with axillary nerve	Supplies huge deltoid muscle, skin overlying it and the shoulder joint

(Contd.)

Table A1.5: Arteries of upper limb (Contd.)

Artery	Origin, course and termination	Area of distribution
Subscapular	Largest branch of axillary artery runs along the muscles of posterior wall of axilla	Supplies muscles of posterior wall of axilla, i.e. teres major, latissimus dorsi, subscapularis. Takes part in anastomoses around scapula
BRACHIAL ARTERY	Starts at the lower border of teres major as continuation of axillary artery. Runs on anterior aspect of arm and ends by dividing into radial and ulnar arteries at neck of radius in the cubital fossa	Supplies muscles of the arm, humerus bone and skin of whole of arm. Takes part in anastomoses around elbow joint
Profunda brachii artery	Largest branch of brachial artery. Runs with radial nerve in the radial sulcus of humerus. Reaching the lateral side of arm ends by dividing into anterior and posterior branches	Supplies muscles of back of arm and its branches anastomose with branches of radial artery and ulnar artery on lateral epicondyle of humerus
Superior ulnar collateral artery	Branch of brachial artery. Accompanies ulnar nerve. Takes part in anastomoses around elbow joint	Supplies muscles of arm and elbow joint on its medial aspect
Muscular branches	Branches arise from brachial artery	Supplies biceps and triceps brachii muscles
Nutrient artery	Branch of brachial and enters the nutrient foramen of humerus	Supplies blood to red bone narrow
Inferior ulnar collateral artery	Branch of brachial	Takes part in the anastomoses around elbow joint from medial side

(Contd.)

Table A1.5: Arteries of upper limb (Contd.)

Artery	Origin, course and termination	Area of distribution
RADIAL ARTERY	Starts as smaller branch of brachial artery, lies on the lateral side of forearm, then in the anatomical snuff box to reach the palm, where it continues as deep palmar arch.	Muscles of lateral side of forearm, including the overlying skin. Gives a branch for completion of superficial palmar arch. Digital branches to thumb and lateral side of index finger
Radial recurrent artery	Branch of radial artery	Supplies elbow joint. Takes part in anastomoses around elbow joint
Muscular branches	Branches of radial artery	Muscles attached to radius, e.g. biceps brachii, pronator teres, pronator quadratus, flexor pollicis longus, flexor digitorum superficialis
Superficial palmar branch	Branch of radial artery in lower part of forearm, before radial artery winds posteriorly	Crosses front of thenar muscles and joins the superficial branch of ulnar artery to complete superficial palmar arch
Dorsal carpal branch	Branch of radial artery as it lies in the anatomical snuff box	Supplies wrist joint
Princeps pollicis artery	Branch of radial artery in palm, runs along thumb	Supplies muscles, tendons, skin and joints in relation to thumb
Radialis indicis artery	Branch of radial A in palm runs along radial side of index finger	Supplies tendons, joints and skin of index finger

(Contd.)

Table A1.5: Arteries of upper limb (*Contd.*)

Artery	Origin, course and termination	Area of distribution
ULNAR ARTERY	Originates as the larger terminal branch of brachial artery at neck of radius. Courses first obliquely in upper one-third and then vertically in lower two-thirds of forearm. Lies superficial to flexor retinaculum and ends by dividing into superficial and deep branches	Gives branches to take part in the anastomoses around elbow joint. Branches supply muscles of front of forearm, back of forearm and nutrient arteries to forearm bones
Anterior and posterior ulnar recurrent arteries	Branches of ulnar artery curve upwards and reach elbow joint	Take part in anastomoses around elbow joint
Common interosseous	Large branch of ulnar artery	Supplies all the muscles of forearm
Branches		
(a) Anterior interosseous artery	Branch of common interosseous artery runs on interosseous membrane	Supplies both the bones of forearm and muscles attached to these bones
(b) Posterior interosseous artery	Branch of common interosseous artery reaches back of forearm	Supplies muscles of back of forearm. Also takes part in anastomoses around elbow joint
Superficial branch	Larger terminal branch of ulnar artery joins superficial palmar branch of radial artery to form superficial palmar arch	Gives branches to tendons in the palm, digital branches along fingers. Also supplies joints and overlying skin
Deep branch	Smaller terminal branch of ulnar A. that joins with the terminal part of radial artery to form the deep palmar arch which lies deep to the long flexor tendons of the palm. It is also proximal to the superficial palmar arch	Branches of deep palmar arch join the digital branches of superficial palmar arch, supplementing the blood supply to the digits or fingers

Boxer's palsy or swimmer's palsy: Serratus anterior causes the movement of protraction. If the long thoracic nerve is injured, the muscle gets paralysed, seen as "winging of scapula". Such a person cannot hit his opponent by that hand. Neither can he make strokes while swimming.

Golfer's elbow/medial epicondylitis: Occurs in golf players. Repeated microtraumas to medial epicondyle causes inflammation of common flexor origin and pain in flexing the wrist.

Waiter's tip or policeman's tip: "taking the tip quietly" Erb-Duchenne paralysis occurs due to involvement of Erb's point. At Erb's point C5, C6 roots join to form upper trunk, two divisions of the trunk arise and two branches, the suprascapular and nerve to subclavius also arise. The arm is adducted and medially rotated while the forearm is pronated and extended.

Wrist drop: Paralysis of radial nerve in axilla or radial sulcus or anterolateral side of lower part of arm or paralysis of its deep branch in cubital fossa leads to wrist drop.

Carpal tunnel syndrome: Median nerve gets compressed under the flexor retinaculum, leading to paralysis of muscles of thenar eminence. It is called 'ape-like hand' There is loss of sensation in lateral 3½ digits including nail beds. Median nerve is the '*eye of the hand*'. There is little clawing of index and middle fingers also.

Cubital tunnel syndrome: Ulnar nerve gets entrapped between two heads of flexor carpi ulnaris muscle, leading to paralysis of medial half of flexor digitorum profundus and muscles of hypothenar eminence, all interossei, adductor pollicis and 3rd and 4th lumbricals. There is clawing of medial two digits, gutters in the hand and loss of hypothenar eminence.

Volkmann's ischaemic contracture: This condition occurs due to fibrosis of the muscles of the forearm, chiefly the flexors. It usually occurs with injury to the brachial artery in supracondylar fractures of humerus.

Dupuytren's contracture: This clinical condition is due to fibrosis of medial part of palmar aponeurosis especially the part reaching the ring and little fingers. The fibrous bands are attached to proximal and middle phalanges and not to distal phalanges. So proximal and middle phalanges are flexed, while distal phalanges remain extended.

Funny bone: Ulnar nerve is palpable in flexed elbow behind the medial epicondyle. Palpating the nerve gives rise to funny sensations on the medial side of forearm. Since medial epicondyle is part of humerus, it is called humerus or funny bone.

Pointing finger: Branch of anterior interosseus nerve to lateral half of flexor digitorum profundus is injured in the middle of the forearm. The index finger is affected the most. It remains extended and keeps pointing forwards (despite the fact that remaining three fingers are pointing towards self).

Complete claw hand: Complete claw hand is due to injury of lower trunk of brachial plexus especially the root, which supplies intrinsic muscles of hand. The injury is called 'Klumpke's paralysis'. The metacarpophalangeal joints are extended while both the interphalangeal joints of all fingers are actually flexed.

Breast: The breast is a frequent site of carcinoma (cancer). Several anatomical facts are of importance in diagnosis and treatment of this condition. Abscess may also form in the breast and may require drainage. The following facts are worthy of note.

Incisions into the breast are usually made radially to avoid cutting the lactiferous ducts.

Cancer cells may infiltrate the suspensory ligaments. The breast then becomes fixed. Contraction of the ligaments can cause retraction or puckering (folding) of the skin.

Infiltration of lactiferous ducts and their consequent fibrosis can cause retraction of the nipple.

Obstruction of superficial lymph vessels by cancer cells may produce oedema of the skin giving rise to an appearance like that of the skin of an orange (*peau d' orange* appearance).

Due to bilateral communications of the lymphatics of the breast across the midline, cancer may spread from one breast to the other.

Because of communications of the lymph vessels with those in the abdomen, cancer of the breast may spread to the liver. Cancer cells may 'drop' into the pelvis especially ovary (Kruckenberg's tumour) producing secondaries there.

Apart from the lymphatics cancer may spread through the veins. In this connection, it is important to know that the veins draining the breast communicate with the vertebral venous plexus of veins. Through these communications cancer can spread to the vertebrae and to the brain.

Blood pressure: The blood pressure is universally recorded by auscultating the brachial artery on the anteromedial aspect of the elbow joint.

Intravenous injection: The median cubital vein is the vein of choice for intravenous injections, for withdrawing blood from donors, and for cardiac catheterisation, because it is fixed by the perforator and does not slip away during piercing.

Intramuscular injection: Intramuscular injections are often given into the deltoid. They should be given in the middle of the muscle to avoid injury to the axillary nerve.

Radial pulse: The radial artery is used for feeling the (arterial) pulse at the wrist. The pulsation can be felt well in this situation because of the presence of the flat radius behind the artery.

Ligaments of Cooper: Fibrous strands extend between skin overlying the breast and the underlying pectoral muscles. These support the gland.

Montgomery's glands: Glands beneath the areola of mammary gland.

Subareolar plexus of Sappy: Lymphatic plexus beneath the areola of the breast.

Lister's tubercle: Dorsal tubercle on lower end of posterior surface of radius. This acts as a pulley for the tendon of extensor pollicis longus.

de Quervain's disease is a thickening of sheath around tendons of abductor pollicis longus and extensor pollicis brevis giving rise to pain on lateral side of wrist.

Section II
Thorax

- Introduction
- Bones and Joints of Thorax
- Wall of Thorax
- Thoracic Cavity and the Pleura
- Lungs
- Mediastinum
- Pericardium and Heart
- Superior Vena Cava, Aorta and Pulmonary Trunk
- Trachea, Oesophagus and Thoracic Duct
- Surface Marking of Thorax
- *Appendix 2*

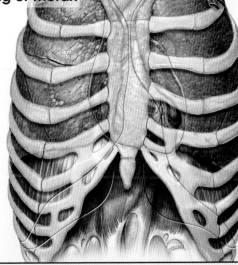

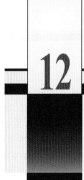

Introduction

Thorax forms the upper part of the trunk of the body. It not only permits boarding and lodging of the thoracic viscera, but also provides necessary shelter to some of the abdominal viscera.

SKELETON OF THORAX

The skeleton of thorax is also known as the thoracic cage. It is an osseocartilaginous, elastic cage which is primarily designed for increasing and decreasing the intrathoracic pressure, so that air is sucked into the lungs during inspiration and expelled during expiration.

Formation

* *Anteriorly* by the sternum
* *Posteriorly* by the 12 thoracic vertebrae and the intervening intervertebral discs.
* *On each side* by 12 ribs with their cartilages.

SUPERIOR APERTURE/INLET OF THORAX

The narrow upper end of the thorax, which is continuous with the neck, is called the inlet of the thorax. It is kidney-shaped. Its transverse diameter is 10–12.5 cm. The anteroposterior diameter is about 5 cm.

Boundaries

* *Anteriorly:* Upper border of the manubrium sterni
* *Posteriorly:* Superior surface of the body of the first thoracic vertebra
* *On each side:* First rib with its cartilage

The plane of the inlet is directed downwards and forwards with an obliquity of about 45 degrees. The anterior part of the inlet lies 3.7 cm below the posterior part, so that the upper border of the manubrium sterni lies at the level of the upper border of the third thoracic vertebra.

Partition at the Inlet of Thorax

The partition is in two halves, right and left, with a cleft in between. Each half is also known as Sibson's fascia or suprapleural membrane. It partly separates the thorax from the neck. The membrane is triangular in shape. Its apex is attached to the tip of the transverse process of the seventh cervical vertebra and the base to the inner border of the first rib and its cartilage. Morphologically it is regarded as the flattened tendon of the scalenus minimus (pleuralis) muscle. Functionally, it provides rigidity to the thoracic inlet, so that the root of the neck is not puffed up and down during respiration. The inferior surface of the membrane is fused to the cervical pleura, beneath which lies the apex of the lung. Its superior surface is related to the subclavian vessels and other structures at the root of the neck (Fig. 12.1).

Structures Passing through the Inlet of Thorax

Viscera

Trachea, oesophagus, apices of the lungs with pleura, remains of the thymus.

Large Vessels

Brachiocephalic artery on right side

Left common carotid artery and the left subclavian artery on the left side. Right and left brachiocephalic veins.

Nerves

• Right and left phrenic nerves
• Right and left vagus nerves

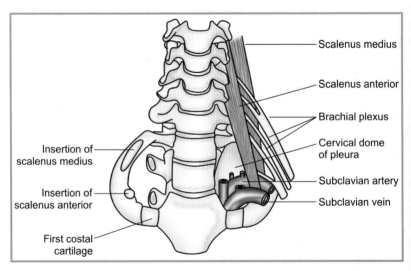

Fig. 12.1: Thoracic inlet showing cervical dome of the pleura on left side of body and its relationship to inner border of first rib.

- Right and left sympathetic trunks
- Right and left first thoracic nerves as they ascend across the first rib to join the brachial plexus.

Muscles

Sternohyoid, sternothyroid and longus colli.

INFERIOR APERTURE/OUTLET OF THORAX

The inferior aperture is the broad end of the thorax which surrounds the upper part of the abdominal cavity but is separated from it by the diaphragm.

Boundaries

- *Anteriorly:* Infrasternal angle between the two costal margins.
- *Posteriorly:* Inferior surface of the body of the twelfth thoracic vertebra.
- *On each side:* Costal margin formed by the cartilages of seventh to twelfth ribs.

Structures Passing through the Diaphragm

There are three large, and several small, openings in the diaphragm which allow passage to structures from thorax to abdomen or *vice versa* (Fig. 12.2).

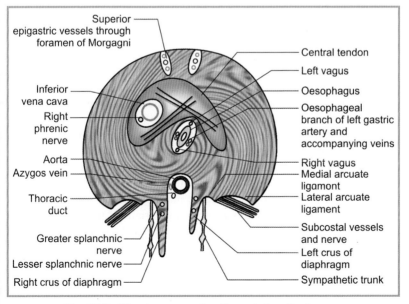

Fig. 12.2: Structures passing through the diaphragm.

Large Openings in the Diaphragm

A. The *aortic opening* is osseoaponeurotic. It lies at the lower border of the twelfth thoracic vertebra. It transmits
   (i) Aorta
   (ii) Thoracic duct
   (iii) Azygos vein

B. The *oesophageal opening* lies in the muscular part of the diaphragm, at the level of the tenth thoracic vertebra. It transmits
   (i) Oesophagus
   (ii) Gastric (vagus) nerves
   (iii) Oesophageal branches of the left gastric artery, with some oesophageal veins that accompany the arteries.

C. The *vena caval opening* lies in the central tendon of the diaphragm at the level of the eighth thoracic vertebra. It transmits
   (i) The inferior vena cava
   (ii) Branches of the right phrenic nerve

CLINICAL ANATOMY

- The chest wall of the child is highly elastic, and fractures of the ribs are, therefore, rare. In adults, the ribs may be fractured by direct or indirect violence. In indirect violence, like crush injury, the rib fractures at its weakest point located at the angle. The upper two ribs which are protected by the clavicle, and the lower two ribs which are free to swing are least commonly injured.

- A cervical rib is a rib attached to vertebra C7. It occurs in about 0.5% of subjects. Such a rib may exert traction on the lower trunk of the brachial plexus which arches over a cervical rib. Such a person complains of paraesthesia or abnormal sensations along the ulnar border of the forearm, and wasting of the small muscles of the hand supplied by segment T1. Vascular changes may also occur.

- In coarctation or narrowing of the aorta, the posterior intercostal arteries get enlarged greatly to provide a collateral circulation. Pressure of the enlarged arteries produces characteristic notching on the ribs..

- *Thoracic inlet syndrome:* Two structures arch over the first rib—the subclavian artery and first thoracic nerve. These structures may be pulled or pressed by a cervical rib or by variations in the insertion of the scalenus anterior. The symptoms may, therefore, be vascular, neural, or both.

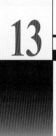

Bones and
Joints of Thorax

BONES OF THORAX

RIBS OR COSTAE

1. There are 12 ribs on each side forming the greater part of the thoracic skeleton.
2. The ribs are bony arches arranged one below the other. The gaps between the ribs are called intercostal spaces.
3. The first 7 ribs which are connected through their cartilages to the sternum are called true ribs, or vertebrosternal ribs. The remaining five are false ribs. Out of these the cartilages of the eighth, ninth and tenth ribs are joined to the next higher cartilage and are known as vertebrochondral ribs. The anterior ends of the eleventh and twelfth ribs are free and are called floating ribs or vertebral ribs.
4. The first two and last three ribs have special features, and are atypical ribs. The third to ninth ribs are typical ribs.

Features of a Typical Rib

Each rib has two ends, anterior and posterior. Its shaft comprises upper and lower borders, and outer and inner surfaces.

The *anterior end* is oval and concave for articulation with its costal cartilage.

The *posterior or vertebral end* is made up of the following parts.

1. The *head* has two facets that are separated by a crest. The lower larger facet articulates with the body of the numerically corresponding vertebra while the upper smaller facet articulates with the next higher vertebra (Fig. 13.1).
2. The *tubercle* is placed on the outer surface of the rib at the junction of the neck and shaft. Its medial part is articular and forms the costotransverse joint with the transverse process of the corresponding vertebra. The lateral part is non-articular.

The *shaft* is flattened so that it has two surfaces, outer and inner; and two borders, upper and lower. The shaft is curved with its convexity

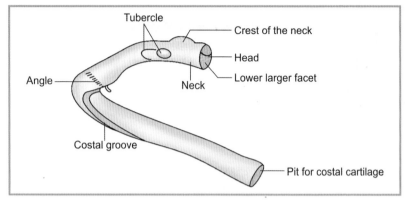

Fig. 13.1: A typical rib viewed obliquely from behind.

outwards (Fig. 13.1). It is bent at the *angle* which is situated about 5 cm lateral to the tubercle. It is also twisted at the angle.

1. The *outer surface:* The angle is marked by an oblique line on the outer surface directed downwards and laterally.
2. The *inner surface* is smooth and covered by the pleura. This surface is marked by a ridge which is continuous behind with the lower border of the neck. The costal groove lies between this ridge and the inferior border. The costal groove contains the posterior intercostal vessels and intercostal nerve.
3. The *upper border* is thick and has outer and inner lips.

First Rib

Identification

1. It is the shortest, broadest and most curved rib.
2. The shaft is not twisted.
3. It is flattened from above downwards so that it has superior and inferior surfaces and outer and inner borders.

Side Determination

1. The anterior end is larger, thicker and pitted. The posterior end is small and rounded.
2. The outer border is convex.
3. The upper surface of the shaft is crossed obliquely by two shallow grooves separated by a ridge. The ridge is enlarged at the inner border of the rib to form the *scalene tubercle.*

Attachments and Relations

1. Anteriorly, the neck is related from medial to lateral side to:
   (i) Sympathetic chain

    (ii) Posterior intercostal vein

   (iii) Posterior intercostal artery

   (iv) First thoracic nerve (Fig. 13.2) (chain pulling a VAN)

2. The anterior groove on the superior surface of the shaft lodges the subclavian vein, and the posterior groove lodges the subclavian artery and the lower trunk of the brachial plexus.

3. The structures attached to the upper surface of the shaft are:

    (i) The origin of the subclavius muscle at the anterior end

   (ii) The attachment of the costoclavicular ligament at the anterior end behind the subclavius

   (iii) The insertion of the scalenus anterior on the scalene tubercle

   (iv) The insertion of the scalenus medius on the elongated rough area behind the groove for the subclavian artery.

Second Rib

Features

The features of the second rib are as follows.

1. The length is twice that of the first rib

2. The shaft has no twist. The outer surface is convex and faces more upwards than outwards. Near its middle it is marked by a large rough tubercle. This tubercle is a unique feature of the second rib. The inner surface of the shaft is smooth and concave. It faces more downwards than inwards. There is a short costal groove on the posterior part of this surface.

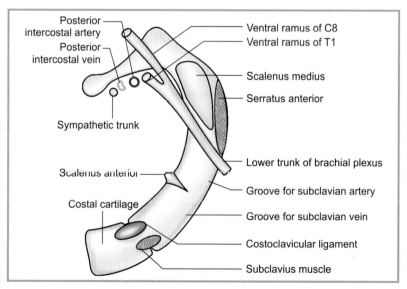

Fig. 13.2: Superior view of the first rib (left side).

Attachments

The rough tubercle on the outer surface gives origin to one and a half digitations of the serratus anterior muscle.

Tenth Rib

The tenth rib closely resembles a typical rib, but is
 (i) Shorter
 (ii) Has only a single facet on the head, for the body of the tenth thoracic vertebra

Eleventh and Twelfth Ribs

Eleventh and twelfth ribs are short. They have pointed ends. The necks and tubercles are absent. The angle and costal groove are poorly marked in the eleventh rib; and are absent in the twelfth rib.

Attachment and Relations of the Twelfth Rib

1. The capsular and radiate ligaments are attached to the head of the rib.
2. The following are attached on the inner surface
    (i) The quadratus lumborum is inserted into the lower part of the medial half to two-thirds of this surface
    (ii) The fascia covering the quadratus lumborum is also attached to this part of the rib
    (iii) The internal intercostal muscle is inserted near the upper border
    (iv) The costodiaphragmatic recess of the pleura is related to the medial three-fourths of the costal surface
    (v) The diaphragm takes origin from the anterior end of this surface
3. The following are attached to the outer surface
    A. Attachments on the medial half
    (i) Costotransverse ligament
    (ii) Lumbocostal ligament
    (iii) Lowest levator costae
    (iv) Iliocostalis and longissimus parts of sacrospinalis.
    B. Attachments on the lateral half
    (i) Insertion of serratus posterior inferior
    (ii) Origin of latissimus dorsi
    (iii) Origin of external oblique muscle of abdomen.
4. The intercostal muscles are attached to the upper border.
5. The structures attached to the lower border are:
    (i) Middle layer of thoracolumbar fascia
    (ii) Lateral arcuate ligament, at the lateral border of the quadratus lumborum
    (iii) Lumbocostal ligament near the head, extending to the transverse process of first lumbar vertebra

STERNUM

The sternum is a flat bone, forming the anterior median part of the thoracic skeleton. In shape, it resembles a short sword. The upper part, corresponding to the handle is called the *manubrium*. The middle part, resembling the blade is called the body. The lowest tapering part forming the point of the sword is the *xiphoid process* or xiphisternum.

The sternum is about 17 cm long. It is longer in males than in females.

Attachments

1. The anterior surface gives origin on either side to
   (i) The pectoralis major
   (ii) The sternal head of the sternocleidomastoid (Fig. 13.3)

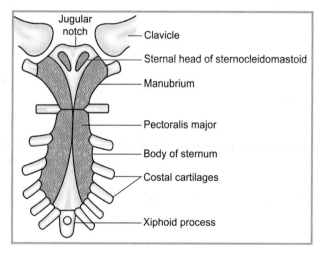

Fig. 13.3: The sternum: Anterior aspect.

2. The posterior surface gives origin to
   (i) The sternohyoid in upper part
   (ii) The sternothyroid in lower part. The lower half of this surface is related to the arch of the aorta. The upper half is related to the left brachiocephalic vein, the brachiocephalic artery, the left common carotid artery and the left subclavian artery. The lateral portions of the surface are related to the corresponding lung and pleura.
3. The suprasternal notch gives attachment to the lower fibres of the interclavicular ligament, and to the two subdivisions of the investing layer of cervical fascia.
4. The margins of each clavicular notch give attachment to the capsule of the corresponding sternoclavicular joint.

Body of the Sternum

The body is longer, narrower and thinner than the manubrium. It is widest close to its lower end opposite the articulation with the fifth costal cartilage. It has two surfaces, anterior and posterior; two lateral borders; and two ends, upper and lower.

1. The *anterior surface* is nearly flat and directed forwards and slightly upwards. It is marked by three ill-defined transverse ridges, indicating the lines of fusion of the four small segments called sternebrae.
2. The posterior surface is slightly concave and is marked by less distinct transverse lines.
3. The lateral borders form synovial joints with the lower part of the second costal cartilage, the third to sixth costal cartilages, and the upper half of the seventh costal cartilage.
4. The upper end forms a secondary cartilaginous joint with the manubrium, at the sternal angle.
5. The lower end is narrow and forms a primary cartilaginous joint with the xiphisternum.

Attachments

1. The anterior surface gives origin on either side to the pectoralis major muscle.
2. The lower part of the posterior surface gives origin on either side to the sternocostalis muscle.
3. On the right side of the median plane, the posterior surface is related to the anterior border of the right lung and pleura. On the left side the upper two pieces of the body are related to the left lung and pleura, and the lower two pieces to the pericardium (Fig. 13.4).

Xiphoid Process

The xiphoid process is the smallest part of the sternum. It is at first cartilaginous, but in the adult it becomes ossified near its upper end. It varies greatly in shape and may be bifid or perforated. It lies in the floor of the epigastric fossa.

Attachments

1. The anterior surface provides insertion to the medial fibres of the rectus abdominis, and to the aponeuroses of the external and internal oblique muscles of the abdomen.
2. The posterior surface gives origin to the diaphragm. It is related to the anterior surface of the liver.
3. The lateral borders of the xiphoid process give attachment to the aponeuroses of the internal oblique and transversus abdominis muscles.
4. The upper end forms a primary cartilaginous joint with the body of the sternum.

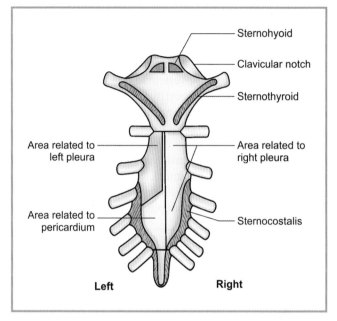

Fig. 13.4: Attachments on the posterior surface of the sternum.

VERTEBRAL COLUMN

Curvatures

In Sagittal Plane

1. *Primary curves* are present at birth due to the shape of the vertebral bodies. The primary curves are thoracic and sacral, both of which are concave forwards.
2. *Secondary curves* are postural and are mainly due to the shape of the intervertebral disc. The secondary or compensatory curves are cervical and lumbar, both of which are convex forwards. The cervical curve appears during four to five months after birth when the infant starts supporting its head: The lumbar curve appears during twelve to eighteen months when the child assumes the upright posture.

In Coronal Plane (lateral curve)

There is slight lateral curve in the thoracic region with its concavity towards the left. It is possible due to the greater use of the right upper limb and the pressure of the aorta.

The curvatures add to the elasticity of the spine, and the number of curves gives it a higher resistance to weight than would be afforded by a single curve.

Parts of a Typical Vertebra

A typical vertebra is made up of the following parts.

1. The *body* lies anteriorly. It is shaped like a short cylinder, being rounded from side to side and having flat upper and lower surfaces that are attached to those of adjoining vertebrae by intervertebral discs.
2. The *pedicles:* right and left are short rounded bars that project backwards, and somewhat laterally, from the posterior aspect of the body.
3. Each pedicle is continuous, posteromedially, with a vertical plate of bone called the *lamina*.
4. Bounded anteriorly by the posterior aspect of the body, on the sides by the pedicles, and behind by the lamina, there is a large *vertebral foramen.*
5. Passing backwards and usually downwards from the junction of the two laminae there is the spine or spinous process (Fig. 13.5).

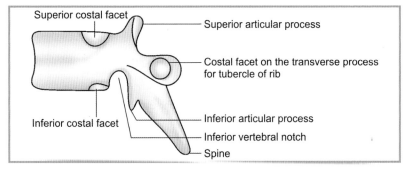

Fig. 13.5: Typical thoracic vertebra, lateral view.

6. Passing laterally and usually somewhat downwards from the junction of each pedicle and the corresponding lamina, there is a *transverse process.*
7. Projecting upwards from the junction of the pedicle and the lamina there is on either side, a *superior articular process;* and projecting downwards there is an *inferior articular process.*
8. The pedicle is much narrower in vertical diameter than the body and is attached nearer its upper border. As a result there is a large *inferior vertebral notch* below the pedicle. Above the pedicle there is a much shallower *superior vertebral notch.*

Thoracic Vertebrae

Identification

The thoracic vertebrae are identified by the presence of costal facets on the sides of the vertebral bodies. The costal facets may be two or only one on each side. There are 12 thoracic vertebrae, out of which the second to eighth are typical, and the remaining five (first, ninth, tenth, eleventh and twelfth) are atypical.

Typical Thoracic Vertebra

A. The body is heart-shaped with roughly the same measurements from side to side and anteroposteriorly.

B. *The vertebral foramen* is comparatively small and circular.

C. *The vertebral arch shows*

1. The *pedicles* are directed straight backwards.
2. The *laminae* overlap each other from above.
3. The *superior articular processes* project upwards from the junction of the pedicles and laminae.
4. The *inferior articular processes* are fused to the laminae.
5. The *transverse processes* are large, and are directed laterally and backwards from the junction of the pedicles and laminae.
6. The *spine* is long, and is directed downwards and backwards. The fifth to ninth spines are the longest, more vertical and overlap each other. The upper and lower spines are less oblique in direction.

First Thoracic Vertebra

1. The body of this vertebra resembles that of a cervical vertebra.
   The superior costal facet on the body is complete. It articulates with the head of the first rib. The inferior costal facet is a 'demifacet' for the second rib.
2. The spine is thick, long and nearly horizontal.

Ninth Thoracic Vertebra

The ninth thoracic vertebra resembles a typical thoracic vertebra except that the body has only the superior costal demifacets. The inferior costal facets are absent.

Tenth Thoracic Vertebra

The tenth thoracic vertebra resembles a typical thoracic vertebra except that the body has a single complete superior costal facet on each side, extending onto the root of the pedicle.

Eleventh Thoracic Vertebrae

1. The body has a single large costal facet on each side, extending onto the upper part of the pedicle.
2. The transverse process is small, and has no articular facet.
   Sometimes it is difficult to differentiate between thoracic tenth and eleventh vertebrae.

Twelfth Thoracic Vertebra

The shape of the body, pedicles, transverse processes and spine are similar to those of a lumbar vertebra. However, the body bears a single costal facet on each side, which lies more on the lower part of the pedicle than on the body.

JOINTS OF THORAX

Manubriosternal Joint

Manubriosternal joint is a secondary cartilaginous joint. It permits slight movements of the body of the sternum on the manubrium during respiration.

Costovertebral Joints

The head of a typical rib articulates with its own vertebra, and also with the body of the next higher vertebra, to form two plane synovial joints separated by an intra-articular ligament.

Costotransverse Joints

The tubercle of a typical rib articulates with the transverse process of the corresponding vertebra to form a synovial joint.

Rotation of rib-neck backwards causes elevation of second to sixth ribs with moving forwards and upwards of the sternum. This increases the anteroposterior diameter of the thorax (Fig. 13.6).

The articular surfaces of the seventh to tenth ribs are flat, permitting up and down gliding movements or bucket-handle movements of the lower ribs. When the neck of seventh to tenth ribs moves upwards, backwards and medially the result is increase in infrasternal angle. This causes increase in transverse diameter of thorax (Fig. 13.7).

Costochondral Joints

Each rib is continuous anteriorly with its cartilage, to form a primary cartilaginous joint. No movements are permitted at these joints.

Chondrosternal Joints

The first chondrosternal joint is a primary cartilaginous joint, it does not permit any movement. This helps in the stability of the shoulder girdle and of the upper limb.

The second to seventh costal cartilages articulate with the sternum by synovial joints. Each joint has a single cavity except in the second joint where the cavity is divided in two parts. The joints are held together by the capsular and radiate ligaments.

Interchondral Joints

The fifth to ninth costal cartilages articulate with one another by synovial joints. The tenth cartilage is united to the ninth by fibrous tissue.

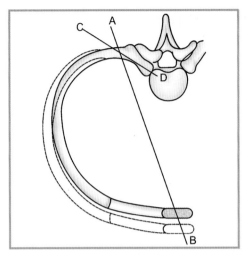

Fig. 13.6: A diagram showing the axes of movement (AB and CD) of a vertebrosternal rib. The interrupted lines indicate the position of the rib in inspiration.

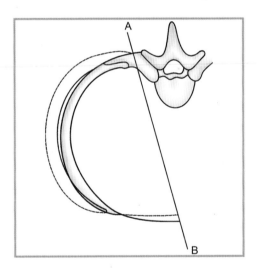

Fig. 13.7: A diagram showing the axes of movement (AB) of a vertebrochondral rib. The interrupted lines indicate the position of the rib in inspiration.

Intervertebral Joints

The joint between the vertebral bodies is a symphysis (secondary cartilaginous joint).

RESPIRATORY MOVEMENTS

The lungs expand during inspiration and retract during expiration. These movements are governed by the following two factors.

(i) Alterations in the capacity of the thorax are brought about by movements of the thoracic wall. Increase in volume of the thoracic cavity creates a negative intrathoracic pressure which sucks air into the lungs. Movements of the thoracic wall occur chiefly at the costovertebral and manubriosternal joints.

(ii) Elastic recoil of the pulmonary alveoli and of the thoracic wall expels air from the lungs during expiration.

Summary of the Factors Producing Increase in Diameters of the Thorax

The anteroposterior diameter is increased:

(i) Mainly by the 'pump-handle' movements of the sternum brought about by elevation of the vertebrosternal second to sixth ribs.

(ii) Partly by elevation of the seventh to tenth vertebrochondral ribs.

The transverse diameter is increased:

(i) Mainly by the 'bucket-handle' movements of the seventh to tenth vertebrochondral ribs.

(ii) Partly by elevation of the second to sixth vertebrosternal ribs.

The vertical diameter is increased by descent of the diaphragm as it contracts.

Respiratory Muscles

1. During quiet breathing, inspiration is brought about chiefly by the diaphragm and partly by the intercostal muscles: Quiet expiration occurs passively by the elastic recoil of the pulmonary alveoli and thoracic wall.

2. During forced breathing, inspiration is brought about by the diaphragm, the intercostal muscles, the sternocleidomastoids, the scaleni, the serratus anterior, the pectoralis minor, and the erector spinae. The alaequae nasi open up the external nares. Forced expiration is brought about by the muscles of the abdominal wall and by the latissimus dorsi.

CLINICAL ANATOMY

- Bone marrow for examination is usually obtained by manubriosternal puncture.
- The slight movements that take place at the manubriosternal joint are essential for movements of the ribs.
- In the anomaly called 'funnel chest', the sternum is depressed.

- In another anomaly called 'pigeon chest', there is forward projection of the sternum like the keel of a boat, and flattening of the chest wall on either side.

- In young adults, the discs are very strong. However, after the second decade of life degenerative changes set in resulting in weakness of the annulus fibrosus. When such a disc is subjected to strain the annulus fibrosus may rupture leading to prolapse of the nucleus pulposus. This is commonly referred to as disc prolapse. It may occur even after a minor strain. In addition to prolapse of the nucleus pulposus, internal derangements of the disc may also take place.

- Disc prolapse is usually posterolateral. The prolapsed nucleus pulposus presses upon adjacent nerve roots and gives rise to pain that radiates along the distribution of the nerve. Such pain along the course of the sciatic nerve is called *sciatica*. Motor effects, with loss of power and reflexes, may follow. Disc prolapse occurs most frequently in the lower lumbar region. It is also common in the lower cervical region from fifth to seventh cervical vertebrae.

- In dyspnoea or difficulty in breathing, the patients are most comfortable on sitting up, leaning forwards and fixing the arms. In the sitting posture, the position of diaphragm is lowest allowing maximum ventilation. Fixation of the arms fixes the scapulae, so that the serratus anterior and pectoralis minor may act on the ribs to good advantage.

- The height of the diaphragm in the thorax is variable according to the position of the body and tone of the abdominal muscles. It is highest on lying supine, so the patient is extremely uncomfortable, as he/she needs to exert immensely for inspiration. The diaphragm is lowest while sitting. The patient is quite comfortable as the effort required for inspiration is the least.

   The diaphragm is midway in position while standing, but the patient is too ill or exhausted to stand. So dyspnoeic patients feel comfortable while sitting.

- Weakest area of rib is the region of its angle. This is the commonest site of fracture.

- For cardiac surgery, the manubrium and/or body of sternum need to be split.

- Sternum is protected from injury by attachment of elastic costal cartilages. Indirect violence may lead to fracture of sternum.

- Cervical rib occurs in 0.5% of persons. It may articulate with first rib or may have a free end. It may cause pressure on lower trunk of brachial plexus, resulting in paraesthesia along the medial border of forearms and wasting of intrinsic muscles of hand. It may also cause pressure on the subclavian artery.

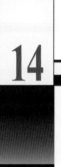

Wall of Thorax

THORACIC WALL PROPER

The thoracic cage forms the skeletal framework of the wall of the thorax. The gaps between the ribs are called intercostal spaces. They are filled by the intercostal muscles and contain the intercostal nerves, vessels and lymphatics.

Intercostal Muscles

These are as follows.
  (i) The external intercostal muscle
 (ii) The internal intercostal muscle
(iii) The transversus thoracis muscle which is divisible into three parts, namely the subcostalis, the intercostalis intimi and the sternocostalis. The attachments of these muscles are given in Table 14.1.

Direction of Fibres

In the anterior part of the intercostal space
1. The fibres of the external intercostal muscle run downwards, forwards and medially.
2. The fibres of the internal intercostal run downwards, backwards and laterally, i.e. at right angle to those of the external intercostal.
3. The fibres of the transversus thoracis run in the same direction as those of the internal intercostal.

Nerve Supply

All intercostal muscles are supplied by the intercostal nerves of the spaces in which they lie.

Actions of the Intercostal Muscles

1. The main action of the intercostal muscles is to prevent intercostal spaces being drawn in during inspiration and from bulging outwards during expiration.
2. The external intercostals, interchondral portions of the internal intercostals, and the levator costae may elevate the ribs during inspiration.

118

Table 14.1: The attachments of the intercostal muscles (Fig. 14.1)

Muscle	Origin	Insertion
1. External intercostal	Lower border of the rib above the space	Outer lip of the upper border of the rib below
2. Internal intercostal	Floor of the costal groove of the rib above	Inner lip of the upper border of the rib below
3. Transversus thoracis		
(a) Subcostalis	Inner surface of the rib near the angle	Inner surface of two or three ribs below
(b) Intercostalis intimi	Middle two-fourths of the ridge above the costal groove	Inner lip of the upper border of the rib below
(c) Sternocostalis	• Lower one-third of the posterior surface of the body of the sternum	Costal cartilages of the 2nd to 6th ribs
	• Posterior surface of the xiphoid	
	• Posterior surface of the costal cartilages of the lower 3 or 4 true ribs near the sternum	

3. The internal intercostals except for the interchondral portions and the transversus thoracis may depress the ribs or cartilages during expiration.

VESSELS AND NERVES

See Appendix 2.

CLINICAL ANATOMY

- Irritation of the intercostal nerves causes severe pain which is referred to the front of the chest or abdomen, i.e. at the peripheral termination of the nerve. This is known as root pain or girdle pain.
- Pus from the vertebral column tends to track around the thorax along the course of the neurovascular bundle and may point at any of the three sites of exit of the branches of a thoracic nerve; one dorsal primary ramus and two cutaneous branches.
- In superior vena caval obstruction, the vena azygos is the main channel which transmits the blood from the upper half of the body to the inferior vena cava.
- Cold abscess occurs due to tubercular infection of the vertebral column. Contents of cold abscess in thoracic region may extend along the course

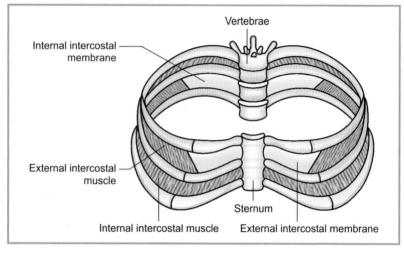

Fig. 14.1: Two layers of a typical intercostal space.

of intercostal nerve. The swelling may present itself at the anterior end of intercostal space or in the anterior abdominal wall. It may present itself in the midaxillary line or on the back along the dorsal ramus of spinal nerve.

• Cardiac pain is an ischaemic pain caused by incomplete obstruction of a coronary artery.

Axons of pain fibres conveyed by the sensory sympathetic cardiac nerves reach thoracic one to thoracic five segments of spinal cord mostly through the dorsal root ganglia of the left side. Since these dorsal root ganglia also receive sensory impulses from the medial side of arm, forearm and upper part of front of chest, the cardiac pain is referred to medial side of left upper limb.

Though the pain is usually referred to the left side, it may even be referred to right arm, jaw, epigastrium or back.

15

Thoracic Cavity and the Pleura

The spongy lungs occupying a major portion of thoracic cavity are enveloped in a serous cavity—the pleural cavity. There is always slight negative pressure in this cavity. During inspiration the pressure becomes more negative, and air is drawn into the lungs covered with its visceral and parietal layers. Visceral layer is inseparable from the lung and is supplied by the same arteries, veins and nerves as lungs. In a similar manner, the parietal pleura follows the walls of the thoracic cavity with cervical, costal, diaphragmatic and mediastinal parts. Pleural cavity limits the expansion of the lungs.

PLEURA

The pleura is a serous membrane which is lined by mesothelium (flattened epithelium). There are two pleural sacs, one on either side of the mediastinum. Each pleural sac is invaginated from its medial side by the lung, so that it has an outer layer, the *parietal pleura,* and an inner layer, the *visceral or pulmonary pleura.*

PULMONARY PLEURA

The serous layer of pulmonary pleura covers the surfaces and fissures of the lung.

PARIETAL PLEURA

The parietal pleura is thicker than the pulmonary pleura, and is subdivided into the following four parts.

  (i) Costal lines thoracic wall
 (ii) Diaphragmatic lines superior aspect of diaphragm
(iii) Mediastinal lines mediastinum
(iv) Cervical covers apex of lung (Fig. 15.1).

  The *costal pleura* lines the thoracic wall which comprises ribs and intercostal spaces to which it is loosely attached by a layer of areola tissue called the endothoracic fascia. The *mediastinal pleura* lines the

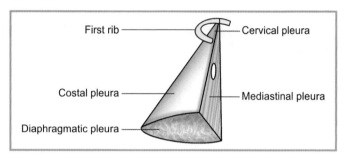

Fig. 15.1: The parietal pleura as a half cone.

corresponding surface of the mediastinum. It is reflected over the root of the lung and becomes continuous with the pulmonary pleura around the hilum. The *cervical pleura* extends into the neck, nearly 5 cm above the first costal cartilage and 2.5 cm above the medial one-third of the clavicle, and covers the apex of the lung. It is covered by the suprapleural membrane. Cervical pleura is related anteriorly to the subclavian artery and the scalenus anterior; posteriorly to the neck of the first rib and structures lying over it; laterally to the scalenus medius; and medially to the large vessels of the neck.

Diaphragmatic pleura lines the superior aspect of diaphragm. It covers the base of the lung and gets continuous with mediastinal pleura medially and costal pleura laterally.

PULMONARY LIGAMENT

The parietal pleura surrounding the root of the lung extends downwards beyond the root as a fold called the pulmonary ligament. The fold contains a thin layer of loose areolar tissue with a few lymphatics. Actually it provides a dead space into which the pulmonary veins can expand during increased venous return as in exercise. The lung roots can also descend into it with the descent of the diaphragm.

RECESSES OF PLEURA

There are two folds or recesses of parietal pleura, which act as 'reserve spaces' for the lung to expand during deep inspiration (Fig. 15.2).

The *costomediastinal recess* lies anteriorly, behind the sternum and costal cartilages, between the costal and mediastinal pleurae, particularly in relation to the cardiac notch of the left lung.

The *costodiaphragmatic recess* lies inferiorly between the costal and diaphragmatic pleura. Vertically it measures about 5 cm, and extends from the eighth to tenth ribs along the midaxillary line.

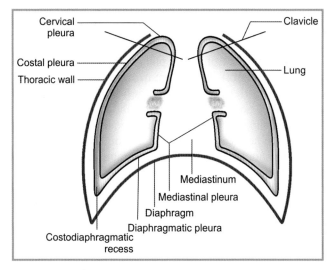

Fig. 15.2: Reflections of pleura as seen in a coronal section of the thorax.

NERVE SUPPLY OF THE PLEURA

The parietal pleura develops from the somatopleuric layer of the lateral plate mesoderm, and is supplied by the somatic nerves. These are the intercostal and phrenic nerves. The parietal pleura is pain sensitive. The costal and peripheral parts of the diaphragmatic pleurae are supplied by the intercostal nerves, and the mediastinal pleura and central part of the diaphragmatic pleurae by the phrenic nerves.

The pulmonary pleura develops from the splanchnopleuric layer of the lateral plate mesoderm, and is supplied by autonomic nerves. The sympathetic nerves are derived from second to fifth spinal segments while parasympathetic nerves are drawn from the vagus nerve.

CLINICAL ANATOMY

- Aspiration of any fluid from the pleural cavity is called *paracentesis thoracis*. It is usually done in the eighth intercostal space in the midaxillary line. The needle is passed through the lower part of the space to avoid injury to the principal neurovascular bundle, i.e. vein, artery and nerve (VAN).
- Some clinical conditions associated with the pleura are as follows.
  (a) *Pleurisy:* This is inflammation of the pleura. It may be dry, but often it is accompanied by collection of fluid in the pleural cavity. The condition is called the pleural effusion.
  (b) *Pneumothorax:* Presence of air in the pleural cavity.

(c) *Haemothorax:* Presence of blood in the pleural cavity

(d) *Hydropneumothorax:* Presence of both fluid and air in the pleural cavity

(e) *Empyema:* Presence of pus in pleural cavity

- Costal and peripheral diaphragmatic pleurae are innervated by intercostal nerves. Hence irritation of these regions cause referred pain along intercostal nerves to thoracic or abdominal wall. Mediastinal and central diaphragmatic pleurae are innervated by phrenic nerve (C4). Hence irritation here causes referred pain on tip of shoulders.
- Pain on right shoulder occurs due to inflammation of gall bladder, while on left shoulder is due to splenic rupture.
- Pleural effusion causes obliteration of costodiaphragmatic recess.

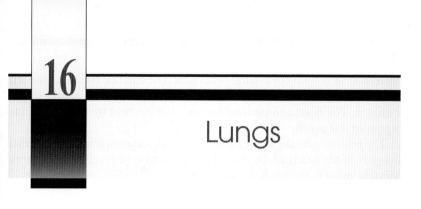

16

Lungs

The lungs are a pair of respiratory organs situated in the thoracic cavity. Each lung invaginates the corresponding pleural cavity. The right and left lungs are separated by the mediastinum.

The lungs are spongy in texture. In the young, the lungs are brown or grey in colour. Gradually, they become mottled black because of the deposition of inhaled carbon particles. The right lung weighs about 700 g; it is about 50–100 g heavier than the left lung.

Features

Each lung is conical in shape (Fig. 16.1). It has
1. An apex at the upper end
2. A base resting on the diaphragm
3. Three borders, i.e. anterior, posterior and inferior
4. Two surfaces, i.e. costal and medial. The medial surface is divided into vertebral and mediastinal parts

The *anterior border* is very thin. It is shorter than the posterior border. On the right side it is vertical and corresponds to the anterior or

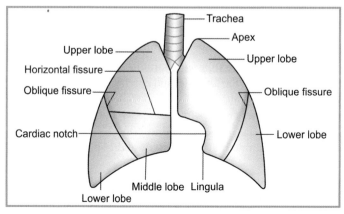

Fig. 16.1: The trachea and lungs as seen from the front.

costomediastinal line of pleural reflection. The anterior border of the left lung shows a wide cardiac notch below the level of the fourth costal cartilage. The heart and pericardium are not covered by the lung in the region of this notch.

The *posterior border* is thick and ill-defined. It corresponds to the medial margins of the heads of the ribs. It extends from the level of the seventh cervical spine to the tenth thoracic spine.

The *inferior border* separates the base from the costal and medial surfaces.

The *costal surface* is large and convex. It is in contact with the costal pleura and the overlying thoracic wall.

The *medial surface* is divided into a posterior or vertebral part, and an anterior or mediastinal part. The vertebral part is related to the vertebral bodies, intervertebral discs, the posterior intercostal vessels and the splanchnic nerves. The mediastinal part is related to the mediastinal septum, and shows a cardiac impression, the hilum and a number of other impressions which differ on the two sides. Various relations of the mediastinal surfaces of the two lungs are listed in Table 16.1.

Fissures and Lobes of the Lungs

The right lung is divided into 3 lobes (upper, middle and lower) by two fissures, oblique and horizontal. The left lung is divided into two lobes by the oblique fissure (Fig. 16.1).

Root of the Lung

Root of the lung is a short, broad pedicle which connects the medial surface of the lung to the mediastinum. It is formed by structures which either enter or come out of the lung at the hilum. The roots of the lungs lie opposite the bodies of the fifth, sixth and seventh thoracic vertebrae.

Contents

The root is made up of the following structures
1. Principal bronchus on the left side, and eparterial and hyparterial bronchi on right side
2. One pulmonary artery
3. Two pulmonary veins, superior and inferior
4. Bronchial arteries, one on the right side and two on the left side
5. Bronchial veins
6. Anterior and posterior pulmonary plexuses of nerves
7. Lymphatics of the lung
8. Bronchopulmonary lymph nodes
9. Areolar tissue

Table 16.1: Structures related to the mediastinal surfaces of the right and left lungs

Right side	Left side
1. Right atrium and auricle	1. Left ventricle, left auricle, infundibulum and adjoining part of the right ventricle
2. A small part of the right ventricle	2. Pulmonary trunk
3. Superior vena cava	3. Arch of aorta
4. Lower part of the right brachiocephalic vein	4. Descending thoracic aorta
5. Azygos vein	5. Left subclavian artery
6. Oesophagus	6. Thoracic duct
7. Inferior vena cava	7. Oesophagus
8. Trachea	8. Left brachiocephalic vein
9. Right vagus nerve	9. Left vagus nerve
10. Right phrenic nerve	10. Left phrenic nerve
	11. Left recurrent laryngeal nerve

Arrangement of Structures in the Root (Fig. 16.2)

A. From before backwards. It is similar on the two sides.
1. Superior pulmonary vein
2. Pulmonary artery
3. Bronchus

B. From above downwards. It is different on the two sides
   Right side
   1. Eparterial bronchus
   2. Pulmonary artery
   3. Hyparterial bronchus
   4. Inferior pulmonary vein
   Left side
   1. Pulmonary artery
   2. Bronchus
   3. Inferior pulmonary vein

Differences Between the Right and Left Lungs

These are given in Table 16.2

Lymphatic Drainage

There are two sets of lymphatics, both of which drain into the broncho-pulmonary nodes.

1. Superficial vessels drain the peripheral lung tissue lying beneath the pulmonary pleura. The vessels pass round the borders of the lung and margins of the fissures to reach the hilum.

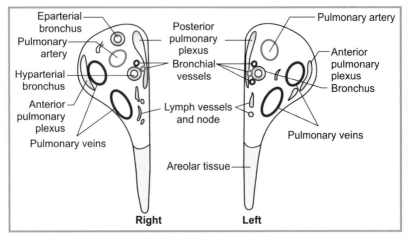

Fig. 16.2: Roots of the right and left lungs seen in section.

Table 16.2: Differences between the right and left lungs

Right lung	Left lung
1. It has 2 fissures and 3 lobes	1. It has only one fissure and 2 lobes
2. Anterior border is straight	2. Anterior border is interrupted by the cardiac notch
3. Larger and heavier, weighs about 700 g	3. Smaller and lighter, weighs about 600 g
4. Shorter and broader	4. Longer and narrower

2. Deep lymphatics drain the bronchial tree, the pulmonary vessels and the connective tissue septa. They run towards the hilum where they drain into the bronchopulmonary nodes.

Nerve Supply

1. Parasympathetic nerves are derived from the vagus. These fibres are:
   (i) Motor to the bronchial muscles, and on stimulation cause bronchospasm
   (ii) Secretomotor to the mucous glands of the bronchial tree
   (iii) Sensory fibres are responsible for the stretch reflex of the lungs and for the cough reflex
2. Sympathetic nerves are derived from second to fifth spinal segments. These are inhibitory to the smooth muscle and glands of the bronchial tree. That is why sympathomimetic drugs, like adrenaline, cause bronchodilatation and relieve symptoms of bronchial asthma.

Both parasympathetic and sympathetic nerves first form anterior and posterior pulmonary plexuses situated in front of and behind the lung roots. From the plexuses nerves are distributed to the lungs along the blood vessels and bronchi.

Bronchial Tree

The *trachea* divides at the level of the lower border of the fourth thoracic vertebra into two primary principal bronchi, one for each lung. The *right principal bronchus* is 2.5 cm long. It is shorter, wider and more in line with the trachea than the left principal bronchus. The *left principal bronchus* is 5 cm long. It is longer, narrower and more oblique than the right bronchus. Right bronchus makes an angle of 25° with tracheal bifurcation, while left bronchus makes an angle of 45° with the trachea.

Each principal bronchus enters the lung through the hilum, and divides into *secondary lobar bronchi,* one for each lobe of the lungs. Thus there are three lobar bronchi on the right side, and only two on the left side. Each lobar bronchus divides into *tertiary or segmental bronchi,* one for each bronchopulmonary segment; which are 10 on the right side and 10 on the left side. The segmental bronchi divide repeatedly to form very small branches called *terminal bronchioles.* Still smaller branches are called *respiratory bronchioles.*

Each respiratory bronchiole aerates a small part of the lung known as a *pulmonary unit.* The respiratory bronchiole ends in microscopic passages which are termed:

(i) Alveolar ducts

(ii) Atria

(iii) Air saccules

(iv) Pulmonary alveoli. Gaseous exchanges take place in the alveoli

Bronchopulmonary Segments

The most widely accepted classification of segments is given in Table 16.3. There are 10 segments on the right side and 10 on the left.

Definition

- These are well-defined anatomic, functional and surgical sectors of the lung
- Each one is aerated by a tertiary or segmental bronchus
- Each segment is pyramidal in shape with its apex directed towards the root of the lung (Fig. 16.3)
- Each segment has a segmental bronchus, segmental artery, autonomic nerves and lymph vessels.

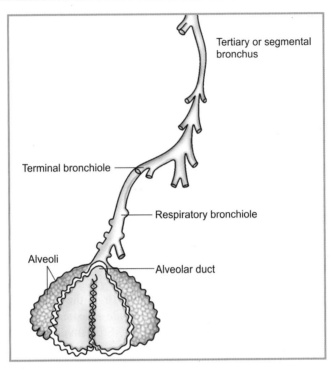

Tertiary or segmental bronchus

Terminal bronchiole

Respiratory bronchiole

Alveoli

Alveolar duct

Fig. 16.3: Diagram of a bronchopulmonary segment.

Table 16.3: The bronchopulmonary segments (Fig. 16.4)

Right lung		Left lung	
Lobes	**Segments**	**Lobes**	**Segments**
A. Upper	1. Apical	A. Upper	1. Apical
	2. Posterior	• Upper division	2. Posterior
	3. Anterior		3. Anterior
B. Middle	4. Lateral	• Lower division	4. Superior lingular
	5. Medial		5. Inferior lingular
C. Lower	6. Superior	B. Lower	6. Superior
	7. Medial basal		7. Medial basal
	8. Anterior basal		8. Anterior basal
	9. Lateral basal		9. Lateral basal
	10. Posterior basal		10. Posterior basal

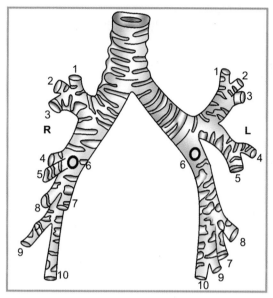

Fig. 16.4: Bronchopulmonary segments of the lungs.

CLINICAL ANATOMY

- Usually the infection of a bronchopulmonary segment remains restricted to it, although tuberculosis and bronchogenic carcinoma may spread from one segment to another.
- Knowledge of the detailed anatomy of the bronchial tree helps considerably in:
  (a) Segmental resection
  (b) Visualising the interior of the bronchi through an instrument passed through the mouth and trachea. The instrument is called a bronchoscope and the procedure is called bronchoscopy
- Carina is the area where trachea divides into two primary bronchi. Right bronchus makes an angle of 25°, while left one makes an angle of 45°. Foreign bodies mostly descend into right bronchus.
- Carina of the trachea is a sensitive area. When patient is made to lie on her/his left side, secretions from right bronchial tree flow towards the carina due to effect of gravity. This stimulates the cough reflex and sputum is brought out. This is called postural drainage.
- Paradoxical respiration: During inspiration the ribs are pulled inside the chest wall while during expiration the ribs seem to be pushed outwards.
- Tuberculosis of lung is one of the commonest diseases. A complete treatment must be taken under the guidance of a physician.

17

Mediastinum

INTRODUCTION

Mediastinum is the middle space left in the thoracic cavity in between the lungs. The mediastinum is the median septum of the thorax between the two lungs. It includes the mediastinal pleurae.

Boundaries

- *Anteriorly*: Sternum
- *Posteriorly*: Vertebral column
- *Superiorly*: Thoracic inlet
- *Inferiorly*: Diaphragm
- *On each side*: Mediastinal pleura

Divisions

For descriptive purposes the mediastinum is divided into the *superior mediastinum* and the *inferior mediastinum.* The inferior mediastinum is further divided into the *anterior, middle and posterior* mediastinum (Fig. 17.1).

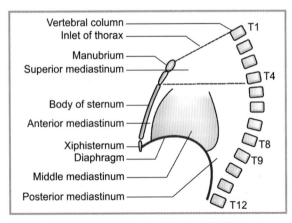

Fig. 17.1: Subdivisions of the mediastinum.

SUPERIOR MEDIASTINUM

Boundaries

- *Anteriorly*: Manubrium sterni
- *Posteriorly*: Upper four thoracic vertebrae
- *Superiorly*: Plane of the thoracic inlet
- *Inferiorly*: An imaginary plane passing through the sternal angle in front, and the lower border of the body of the fourth thoracic vertebra behind
- *On each side*: Mediastinal pleura

Contents

1. Trachea and oesophagus
2. *Muscles:* Origins of (i) sternohyoid, (ii) sternothyroid, (iii) lower ends of longus colli
3. *Arteries:* (i) Arch of aorta, (ii) brachiocephalic artery, (iii) left common carotid artery, (iv) left subclavian artery
4. *Veins:* (i) Right and left brachiocephalic veins, (ii) upper half of the superior vena cava, (iii) left superior intercostal vein
5. *Nerves:* (i) Vagus, (ii) phrenic, (iii) cardiac nerves of both sides, (iv) left recurrent laryngeal nerve
6. Thymus
7. Thoracic duct
8. *Lymph nodes:* Paratracheal, brachiocephalic, and tracheobronchial

INFERIOR MEDIASTINUM

The inferior mediastinum is divided into anterior, middle and posterior mediastina. These are as follows.

Anterior Mediastinum

Anterior mediastinum is a very narrow space in front of the pericardium, overlapped by the thin anterior borders of both lungs. It is continuous through the superior mediastinum with the pretracheal space of the neck.

Contents

  (i) Sternopericardial ligaments
 (ii) Lymph nodes with lymphatics
(iii) Small mediastinal branches of the internal thoracic artery
 (iv) The lowest part of the thymus
  (v) Areolar tissue

Middle Mediastinum

Middle mediastinum is occupied by the pericardium and its contents, along with the phrenic nerves and the pericardiophrenic vessels.

Contents

1. *Heart* enclosed in pericardium
2. *Arteries:* (i) Ascending aorta, (ii) pulmonary trunk, (iii) two pulmonary arteries
3. *Veins:* (i) Lower half of the superior vena cava, (ii) terminal part of the azygos vein, (iii) right and left pulmonary veins
4. *Nerves:* (i) Phrenic, (ii) deep cardiac plexus
5. *Lymph nodes:* Tracheobronchial nodes
6. *Tubes:* (i) Bifurcation of trachea, (ii) the right and left principal bronchi.

Posterior Mediastinum

Contents

1. Oesophagus
2. *Arteries:* Descending thoracic aorta and its branches
3. *Veins:* (i) Azygos vein, (ii) hemiazygos vein, (iii) accessory hemiazygos vein
4. *Nerves:* (i) Vagi, (ii) splanchnic nerves, greater, lesser and least, arising from the lower eight thoracic ganglia of the sympathetic chain
5. *Lymph nodes and lymphatics*
    (i) Posterior mediastinal lymph nodes lying along side the aorta
    (ii) The thoracic duct

CLINICAL ANATOMY

- The prevertebral layer of the deep cervical fascia extends to the superior mediastinum, and is attached to the fourth thoracic vertebra. An infection present in the neck behind this fascia can pass down into the superior mediastinum but not lower down.

    The pretracheal fascia of the neck also extends to the superior mediastinum, where it blends with the arch of the aorta. Neck infections between the pretracheal and prevertebral fasciae can spread into the superior mediastinum, and through it into the posterior mediastinum. Thus mediastinitis can result from infections in the neck.
- There is very little loose connective tissue between the mobile organs of the mediastinum. Therefore, the space can be readily dilated by inflammatory fluids, neoplasms, etc.
- In the superior mediastinum, all large veins are on the right side and the arteries on the left side. During increased blood flow veins expand enormously, while the large arteries do not expand at all. Thus there is much 'dead space' on the right side and it is into this space that tumour or fluids of the mediastinum tend to project.
- The posterior mediastinum is continuous through the superior mediastinum with the neck between the pretracheal and prevertebral

layers of the cervical fascia. This region of the neck includes the retropharyngeal space, spaces on each side of the trachea and oesophagus, the space between these tubes and the carotid sheaths. Infections leading to fluid collections from these spaces can spread to the superior and posterior mediastina.

- Compression of mediastinal structures by any tumour gives rise to a group of symptoms known as *mediastinal syndrome*. The common symptoms are as follows.
  (a) Obstruction of superior vena cava gives rise to engorgement of veins in the upper half of the body
  (b) Pressure over the trachea causes dyspnoea, and cough
  (c) Pressure on oesophagus causes dysphagia
  (d) Pressure or the left recurrent laryngeal nerve gives rise to hoarseness of voice (dysphonia)
  (e) Pressure on the phrenic nerve causes paralysis of the diaphragm on that side
  (f) Pressure on the intercostal nerves gives rise to pain in the area supplied by them. It is called intercostal neuralgia
  (g) Pressure on the vertebral column may cause erosion of the vertebral bodies

The common causes of mediastinal syndrome are bronchogenic carcinoma, Hodgkin's disease causing enlargement of the mediastinal lymph nodes, aneurysm or dilatation of the aorta, etc.

18

Pericardium and Heart

PERICARDIUM

The pericardium is a fibroserous sac which encloses the heart and the roots of the great vessels. It is situated in the middle mediastinum. It consists of the *fibrous pericardium* and the *serous pericardium* (Fig. 18.1).

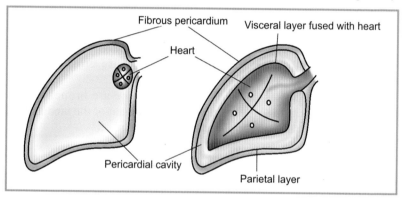

Fibrous pericardium   Visceral layer fused with heart

Heart

Pericardial cavity

Parietal layer

Fig. 18.1: Development of the layers of serous pericardium.

Fibrous pericardium encloses the heart and fuses with the vessels which enter/leave the heart. Heart is situated within the fibrous and serous pericardial sacs. As heart develops, it invaginates itself into the serous sac, without causing any breach in its continuity, the last part to enter is the region of atria, from where the visceral pericardium is reflected as the parietal pericardium. Thus parietal layer of serous pericardium gets adherent to the inner surface of fibrous pericardium, while the visceral layer of serous pericardium gets adherent to the outer layer of heart and forms its epicardium.

FIBROUS PERICARDIUM

Fibrous pericardium is a conical sac made up of fibrous tissue. The parietal layer of serous pericardium is attached to its deep surface.

Serous Pericardium

The *pericardial cavity* is a potential space between the parietal peri-cardium and the visceral pericardium. It contains only a thin film of serous fluid which lubricates the apposed surfaces and allows the heart to beat smoothly.

Sinuses of Pericardium

The *transverse sinus* is a horizontal gap between the arterial and venous ends of the heart tube. It is bounded anteriorly by the ascending aorta and pulmonary trunk, and posteriorly by the superior vena cava and inferiorly by the left atrium. On each side it opens into the general pericardial cavity (Fig. 18.2).

The *oblique sinus* is a narrow gap behind the heart. It is bounded anteriorly by the left atrium, and posteriorly by the parietal pericardium. On the right and left sides it is bounded by reflections of pericardium as shown in Fig. 18.2. Below, and to the left it opens into the rest of the pericardial cavity. The oblique sinus permits pulsations of the left atrium to take place freely (Fig. 18.2).

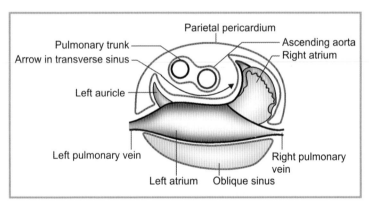

Fig. 18.2: Transverse section through the upper part of the heart. Note the reflections of pericardium, and the mode of formation of the transverse and oblique sinuses.

Contents of the Pericardium

(i) Heart with cardiac vessels and nerves
(ii) Ascending aorta
(iii) Pulmonary trunk
(iv) Lower half of the superior vena cava
(v) Terminal part of the inferior vena cava
(vi) The terminal parts of the pulmonary veins.

Nerve Supply

The fibrous and parietal pericardia are supplied by the phrenic nerve. They are sensitive to pain. The epicardium is supplied by autonomic nerves of the heart, and is not sensitive to pain. Pain of pericarditis originates in the parietal pericardium alone. On the other hand cardiac pain or angina originates in the cardiac muscle or in the vessels of the heart.

HEART

The heart is a conical hollow muscular organ situated in the middle mediastinum. It is enclosed within the pericardium. It pumps blood to various parts of the body to meet their nutritive requirements. The Greek name for the heart is *cardia* from which we have the adjective *cardia*. The Latin name for the heart is *cor* from which we have the adjective *coronary*.

The heart is placed obliquely behind the body of the sternum and adjoining parts of the costal cartilages, so that one-third of it lies to the right and two-thirds to the left of the median plane. The direction of blood flow, from atria to the ventricles is downwards, forwards and to the left. The heart measures about 12 × 9 cm and weighs about 300 g in males and 250 g in females.

External Features

The human heart has four chambers. These are the right and left atria and the right and left ventricles (Fig. 18.3).

The heart has an apex directed downwards, forwards and to the left, a base (or posterior surface) directed backwards; and anterior, inferior and left surfaces.

Grooves or Sulci

The atria are separated from the ventricles by a circular *atrioventricular or coronary sulcus*. The *interatrial groove* is faintly visible posteriorly, while anteriorly it is hidden by the aorta and pulmonary trunk. The *anterior interventricular groove* is nearer to the left margin of the heart. It runs downwards and to the left. The *posterior interventricular groove* is situated on the diaphragmatic or inferior surface of the heart.

Apex of the Heart

Apex of the heart is formed entirely by the left ventricle. It is directed downwards, forwards and to the left and is overlapped by the anterior border of the left lung. It is situated in the left fifth intercostal space 9 cm lateral to the midsternal line just medial to the midclavicular line. In the living subject, pulsations may be seen and felt over this region.

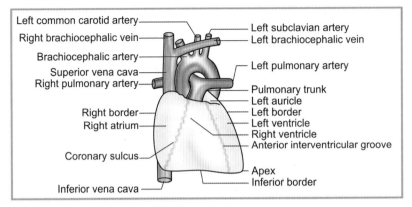

Fig. 18.3: Gross features: Sternocostal surface of heart.

Base of the Heart

The base of the heart is also called its posterior surface. It is formed mainly by the left atrium and by a small part of the right atrium.

Borders of the Heart

The *upper border* is slightly oblique, and is formed by the two atria, chiefly the left atrium. The *right border* is more or less vertical and is formed by the right atrium. The *inferior border* is nearly horizontal and is formed mainly by the right ventricle. A small part of it near the apex is formed by left ventricle. The *left border* is oblique and curved. It is formed mainly by the left ventricle, and partly by the left auricle.

Surfaces of the Heart

The *anterior or sternocostal surface* is formed mainly by the right atrium and right ventricle, and partly by the left ventricle and left auricle.

The *inferior or diaphragmatic surface* rests on the central tendon of the diaphragm. It is formed in its left two-thirds by the left ventricle, and in its right one-third by the right ventricle. It is traversed by the posterior interventricular groove, and is directed downwards and slightly backwards: The *left surface* is formed mostly by the left ventricle, and at the upper end by the left auricle.

RIGHT ATRIUM

The right atrium is the right upper chamber of the heart. It receives venous blood from the whole body, pumps it to the right ventricle through the right atrioventricular or tricuspid opening. It forms the right border, part of the upper border, the sternocostal surface and the base of the heart.

External Features

1. The chamber is elongated vertically, receiving the superior vena cava at the upper end and the inferior vena cava at the lower end (Fig. 18.3).
2. The upper end is prolonged to the left to form the right *auricle.*
3. Along the right border of the atrium there is a shallow vertical groove which passes from the superior vena cava above to the inferior vena cava below. This groove is called the *sulcus terminalis.* It is produced by an internal muscular ridge called the *crista terminalis.* The upper part of the sulcus contains the *sinuatrial or SA node* which acts as the pacemaker of the heart.
4. The right atrioventricular groove separates the right atrium from the right ventricle. It is more or less vertical and lodges the right coronary artery and the small cardiac vein.

Tributaries or Inlets of the Right Atrium

  (i) Superior vena cava
 (ii) Inferior vena cava
(iii) Coronary sinus
(iv) Anterior cardiac veins
 (v) Venae cordis minimi (Thebesian veins)
(vi) Sometimes the right marginal vein

Right Atrioventricular Orifice

Blood passes out of the right atrium through the right atrioventricular or tricuspid orifice and goes to the right ventricle. The tricuspid orifice is guarded by the tricuspid valve which maintains unidirectional flow of blood (Fig. 18.4).

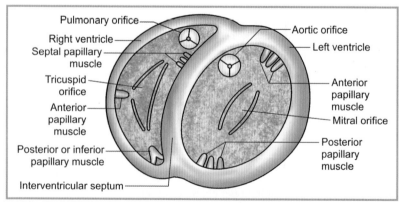

Fig. 18.4: Schematic transverse section through the ventricles of the heart showing the atrioventricular orifices, papillary muscles, and the pulmonary and aortic orifices.

Internal Features

The interior of the right atrium can be broadly divided into three parts.

Smooth Posterior Part or Sinus Venarum

(i) The *superior vena cava* opens at the upper end

(ii) The *inferior vena cava* opens at the lower end

(iii) The *coronary sinus* opens between the opening of the inferior vena cava and the right atrioventricular orifice. The opening is guarded by the *valve of the coronary sinus.*

Rough Anterior Part or Pectinate Part, including the Auricle

1. Developmentally it is derived from the primitive atrial chamber
2. It presents a series of transverse muscular ridges called *musculi pectinati.*

Interatrial Septum

1. It presents the *fossa ovalis*, a shallow saucer-shaped depression, in the lower part.
2. The *annulus ovalis or limbus fossa ovalis* is the prominent margin of the fossa ovalis
3. The remains of the *foramen ovale* are occasionally present.

RIGHT VENTRICLE

The right ventricle is a triangular chamber which receives blood from the right atrium and pumps it to the lungs through the pulmonary trunk and pulmonary arteries. It forms the inferior border and a large part of the sternocostal surface of the heart (Fig. 18.3).

Features

1. Externally, the right ventricle has two surfaces—anterior or sternocostal and inferior diaphragmatic.
2. The interior has two parts
   (i) The *inflowing part* is rough due to the presence of muscular ridges called *trabeculae carneae.*
   (ii) The *outflowing part or infundibulum* is smooth and forms the upper conical part of the right ventricle which gives rise to the pulmonary trunk.
3. The interior shows two orifices
   (i) The right atrioventricular or tricuspid orifice, guarded by the tricuspid valve
   (ii) The pulmonary orifice guarded by the pulmonary valve (Fig. 18.4)
4. The interior of the inflowing part shows *trabeculae carneae or* muscular ridges of three types

   (i) *Ridges* or fixed elevations

  (ii) *Bridges*

 (iii) *Pillars* or papillary muscles with one end attached to the ventricular wall, and the other end connected to the cusps of the tricuspid valve by chordae tendinae. There are three papillary muscles in the right ventricle, anterior, posterior and septal. Each papillary muscle is attached by chordae to the contiguous sides of two cusps.

5. The septomarginal trabecula or moderator band is a muscular ridge extending from the ventricular septum to the base of the anterior papillary muscle. It contains the right branch of the AV bundle.

6. The cavity of the right ventricle is crescentic in section because of the forward bulge of the interventricular septum (Fig. 18.4).

7. The wall of the right ventricle is thinner than that of the left ventricle in a ratio of 1:3.

LEFT ATRIUM

The left atrium is a quadrangular chamber situated posteriorly. Its appendage, the left auricle projects anteriorly to overlap the infundibulum of the right ventricle. The left atrium forms the left two-thirds of the base of the heart, the greater part of the upper border, parts of the sternocostal and left surfaces and of the left border. It receives oxygenated blood from the lungs through four pulmonary veins, and pumps it to the left ventricle through the left atrioventricular or bicuspid or mitral orifice which is guarded by the valve of the same name.

Features

1. The posterior surface of the atrium forms the anterior wall of the oblique sinus of pericardium

2. The anterior wall of the atrium is formed by the interatrial septum

3. Two pulmonary veins open into the atrium on each side of the posterior wall

4. The greater part of the interior of the atrium is smooth walled

LEFT VENTRICLE

The left ventricle receives oxygenated blood from the left atrium and pumps it into the aorta. It forms the apex of the heart, a part of the sternocostal surface, most of the left border and left surface, and the left two-thirds of the diaphragmatic surface.

Features

1. Externally, the left ventricle has three surfaces—anterior or sternocostal, inferior or diaphragmatic, and left.

2. The interior is divisible into two parts
   (i) The lower rough part with trabeculae carneae develops from the primitive ventricle of the heart tube
   (ii) The upper smooth part or aortic vestibule gives origin to the ascending aorta
3. The interior of the ventricle shows two orifices
   (i) The left atrioventricular or bicuspid or mitral orifice, guarded by the bicuspid or mitral valve
   (ii) The aortic orifice, guarded by the aortic valve
4. There are two well-developed papillary muscles, anterior and posterior. Chordae tendinae from both muscles are attached to both the cusps of the mitral valve.
5. The cavity of the left ventricle is circular in cross-section
6. The walls of the left ventricle are three times thicker than those of the right ventricle.

VALVES OF HEART

The valves of the heart maintain unidirectional flow of the blood and prevent its regurgitation in the opposite direction. There are two pairs of valves in the heart, a pair of atrioventricular valves and a pair of semilunar valves. The right atrioventricular valve is known as the tricuspid valve because it has three cusps. The left atrioventricular valve is known as the bicuspid valve because it has two cusps. It is also called the mitral valve. The semilunar valves include the aortic and pulmonary valves, each having three semilunar cusps. The cusps are folds of endocardium, strengthened by an intervening layer of fibrous tissue.

CONDUCTING SYSTEM

The conducting system is made up of myocardium that is specialised for initiation and conduction of the cardiac impulse. Its fibres are finer than other myocardial fibres, and are completely cross-striated. The conducting system has the following parts.
1. **Sinuatrial node or SA node:** It is known as the 'pacemaker' of the heart. It generates an impulse at the rate of about 70/min and initiates the heart beat.
2. **Atrioventricular node or AV node:** It is smaller than the SA node and is situated in the lower and dorsal part of the atrial septum just above the opening of the coronary sinus.
3. **Atrioventricular bundle or AV bundle or bundle of His:** It is the only muscular connection between the atrial and ventricular musculatures. It begins as the atrioventricular (AV) node crosses AV ring and descends along the posteroinferior border of the membranous

part of the ventricular septum. At the upper border of the muscular part of the septum it divides into right and left branches.

4. **The right branch** of the AV bundle passes down the right side of the interventricular septum.

5. **The left branch** of the AV bundle descends on the left side of the interventricular septum and is distributed to the left ventricle after dividing into Purkinje fibres.

6. **The Purkinje fibres** form a subendocardial plexus. They are large pale fibres striated only at their margins. They usually possess double nuclei.

ARTERIES SUPPLYING THE HEART

The heart is supplied by two coronary arteries, arising from the ascending aorta. Both arteries run in the coronary sulcus.

Right Coronary Artery

Right coronary artery is smaller than the left coronary artery. It arises from the anterior aortic sinus (*see* Appendix 2 and Table A2.2).

Left Coronary Artery

Left coronary artery is larger than the right coronary artery. It arises from the left posterior aortic sinus (Fig. 18.5).

VEINS OF THE HEART

These are the great cardiac vein, the middle cardiac vein, the right marginal vein, the posterior vein of the left ventricle, the oblique vein of the left

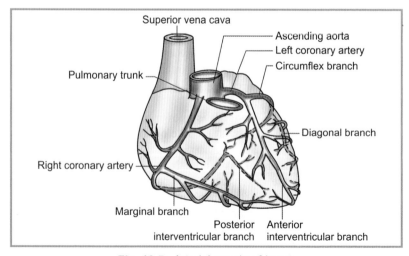

Fig. 18.5: Arterial supply of heart.

atrium, the right marginal vein, the anterior cardiac veins, and the venae cordis minimi. All veins except the last two drain into the coronary sinus which opens into the right atrium. The anterior cardiac veins and the venae cordis minimi open directly into the right atrium.

Coronary Sinus

The coronary sinus is the largest vein of the heart. It is situated in the left posterior coronary sulcus. It is about 3 cm long. It ends by opening into the posterior wall of the right atrium. It receives the following tributaries.
1. Great cardiac vein
2. Middle cardiac vein
3. Small cardiac vein
4. Posterior vein of the left ventricle
5. Oblique vein of the left atrium of Marshall
6. Right marginal vein

Anterior Cardiac Veins

The *anterior cardiac veins* are three or four small veins which run parallel to one another on the anterior wall of the right ventricle and usually open directly into the right atrium through its anterior wall.

Venae Cordis Minimi

The *venae cordis minimi* or *thebesian veins* or *smallest cardiac veins* are numerous small veins present in all four chambers of the heart which open directly into the cavity. These are more numerous on the right side of the heart than on the left. This may be one reason why left sided infarcts are more common.

NERVE SUPPLY OF HEART

Parasympathetic nerves reach the heart via the vagus. These are cardioinhibitory; on stimulation they slow down the heart rate. Sympathetic nerves are derived from the upper four to five thoracic segments of the spinal cord. These are cardioacceleratory, and on stimulation they increase the heart rate, and also dilate the coronary arteries. Both parasympathetic and sympathetic nerves form the superficial and deep cardiac plexuses, the branches of which run along the coronary arteries to reach the myocardium.

The *superficial cardiac plexus* is situated below the arch of the aorta in front of the right pulmonary artery. It is formed by:

(i) The superior cervical cardiac branch of the left sympathetic chain.
(ii) The inferior cervical cardiac branch of the left vagus nerve. It gives branches to the deep cardiac plexus, the right coronary artery, and to the left anterior pulmonary plexus.

The *deep cardiac plexus* is situated in front of the bifurcation of the trachea, and behind the arch of the aorta. It is formed by all the cardiac branches derived from all the cervical and upper thoracic ganglia of the sympathetic chain, and the cardiac branches of the vagus and recurrent laryngeal nerves, except those which form the superficial plexus. The right and left halves of the plexus distribute branches to the corresponding coronary and pulmonary plexuses. Separate branches are given to the atria.

CLINICAL ANATOMY

- Collection of fluid in the pericardial cavity is referred to as pericardial effusion. Pericardial effusion can be drained by puncturing the left fifth or sixth intercostal space just lateral to the sternum, or in the angle between the xiphoid process and left costal margin, with the needle directed upwards, backwards and to the left.
- The first heart sound is produced by closure of the atrioventricular valves. The second heart sound is produced by closure of the semilunar valves.
- Narrowing of the valve orifice due to fusion of the cusps is known as 'stenosis', viz. mitral stenosis, aortic stenosis, etc.
- Dilatation of the valve orifice, or stiffening of the cusps causes imperfect closure of the valve leading to back flow of blood. This is known as incompetence or regurgitation, e.g. aortic incompetence or aortic regurgitation.
- Thrombosis of a coronary artery is a common cause of sudden death in persons past middle age. This is due to myocardial infarction and ventricular fibrillation.
- Incomplete obstruction, usually due to spasm of the coronary artery causes angina pectoris, which is associated with agonising pain in the precordial region and down the medial side of the left arm and forearm. Pain gets relieved by putting appropriate tablets below the tongue.
- Coronary angiography determines the site(s) of narrowing or occlusion of the coronary arteries or their branches.
- Angioplasty helps in removal of small blockage. It is done using small stent or small inflated balloon through a catheter passed upwards through femoral artery, aorta into the coronary artery.
- If there are large segments or multiple sites of blockage, coronary bypass is done using either great saphenous vein or internal thoracic artery as graft(s).
- The area of the chest wall overlying the heart is called the *precordium*
- Rapid pulse or increased heart rate is called *tachycardia*
- Slow pulse or decreased heart rate is called *bradycardia*
- Irregular pulse or irregular heart rate is called *arrhythmia*

- Consciousness of one's heart beat is called *palpitation*
- Inflammation of the heart can involve more than one layer of the heart. Inflammation of the pericardium is called *pericarditis;* of the myocardium is *myocarditis;* and of the endocardium is *endocarditis.*
- Normally the diastolic pressure in ventricles is zero. A positive diastolic pressure in the ventricle is evidence of its failure. Any one of the four chambers of the heart can fail separately, but ultimately the rising back pressure causes right sided failure (congestive cardiac failure or CCF) which is associated with increased venous pressure, oedema on feet, and breathlessness on exertion. Heart failure (right sided) due to lung disease is known as *cor pulmonale.*
- Normally the cardiac apex or apex beat is on the left side. In the condition called dextrocardia, the apex is on the right side. Dextrocardia may be part of a condition called *situs inversus* in which all thoracic and abdominal viscera are a mirror image of normal.
- Cardiac pain is an ischaemic pain caused by incomplete obstruction of a coronary artery.

  Axons of pain fibres conveyed by the sensory sympathetic cardiac nerves reach thoracic one to thoracic five segments of spinal cord mostly through the dorsal root ganglia of the left side. Since these dorsal root ganglia also receive sensory impulses from the medial side of arm, forearm and upper part of front of chest, the pain gets referred to these areas.

  Though the pain is usually referred to the left side, it may even be referred to right arm, jaw, epigastrium or back.

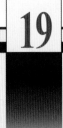

19

Superior Vena Cava, Aorta and Pulmonary Trunk

SUPERIOR VENA CAVA

Superior vena cava is a large venous channel which collects blood from the upper half of the body and drains it into the right atrium. It is formed by the union of the right and left brachiocephalic or innominate veins behind the lower border of the first right costal cartilage close to the sternum. Each brachiocephalic vein is formed behind the corresponding sternoclavicular joint by the union of the internal jugular and subclavian veins.

Course

The superior vena cava is about 7 cm long. It begins behind the lower border of the sternal end of the first right costal cartilage, pierces the pericardium opposite the second right costal cartilage, and terminates by opening into the upper part of the right atrium behind the third right costal cartilage. It has no valves.

AORTA

The aorta is the great arterial trunk which receives oxygenated blood from the left ventricle and distributes it to all parts of the body.

Arch of the Aorta

Arch of the aorta is the continuation of the ascending aorta. It is situated in the superior mediastinum behind the lower half of the manubrium sterni.

Relations

Anteriorly and to the Left

1. Four nerves from before backwards
    (i) Left phrenic
    (ii) Lower cervical cardiac branch of the left vagus
    (iii) Upper cervical cardiac branch of left sympathetic chain
    (iv) Left vagus
2. Left superior intercostal vein, deep to the phrenic nerve and superficial to the vagus nerve

3. Left pleura and lung
4. Remains of thymus

Posteriorly and to the Right

1. Trachea, with the deep cardiac plexus and the tracheobronchial lymph nodes
2. Oesophagus
3. Left recurrent laryngeal nerve
4. Thoracic duct
5. Vertebral column

Superior

1. Three branches of the arch of the aorta
   (i) Brachiocephalic   (ii) Left common carotid
   (iii) Left subclavian
2. All three arteries are crossed close to their origin by the left brachiocephalic vein.

Inferior

1. Bifurcation of the pulmonary trunk
2. Left bronchus
3. Ligamentum arteriosum with superficial cardiac plexus on it
4. Left recurrent laryngeal nerve

DESCENDING THORACIC AORTA

Descending thoracic aorta is the continuation of the arch of the aorta. It lies in the posterior mediastinum (*see* Appendix 2).

PULMONARY TRUNK

The wide pulmonary trunk starts from the summit of infundibulum of right ventricle. Both the ascending aorta and pulmonary trunk are enclosed in a common sleeve of serous pericardium, in front of transverse sinus of pericardium. Pulmonary trunk carrying deoxygenated blood, overlies the beginning of ascending aorta. It courses to the left and divides into right and left pulmonary arteries under the concavity of aortic arch at the level of sternal angle.

The right pulmonary artery courses to the right behind ascending aorta, and superior vena cava and anterior to oesophagus to become part of the root of the lung. It gives off its first branch to the upper lobe before entering the hilum. Within the lung the artery descends posterolateral to the main bronchus and divides like the bronchi into lobar and segmental arteries.

The left pulmonary artery passes to the left anterior to descending thoracic aorta to become part of the root of the left lung. At its beginning, it is connected to the inferior aspect of arch of aorta by ligamentum arteriosus, a remnant of ductus arteriosus. Rest of the course is same as of the right branch.

CLINICAL ANATOMY

- When the superior vena cava is obstructed above the opening of the azygos vein, the venous blood of the upper half of the body is returned through the azygos vein; and the superficial veins are dilated on the chest up to the costal margin.
- When the superior vena cava is obstructed below the opening of the azygos veins, the blood is returned through the inferior vena cava via the femoral vein; and the superior veins are dilated on both the chest and abdomen up to the saphenous opening in the thigh. The superficial vein connecting the lateral thoracic vein with the superficial epigastric vein is known as the *thoracoepigastric* vein.
- In cases of mediastinal syndrome, the signs of superior vena caval obstruction are the first to appear.
- *Aortic knuckle.* In PA view of radiographs of the chest, the arch of the aorta is seen as a projection beyond the left margin of the mediastinal shadow. The projection is called the aortic knuckle. It becomes prominent in old age.
- *Coarctation of the aorta* is a localised narrowing of the aorta opposite to or just beyond the attachment of the ductus arteriosus. An extensive collateral circulation develops between the branches of the subclavian arteries and those of the descending aorta. These include the anastomoses between the anterior and posterior intercostal arteries. These arteries enlarge greatly and produce a characteristic notching on the ribs.
- *Ductus arteriosus, ligamentum arteriosum and patent ductus arteriosus:* During foetal life, the *ductus arteriosus* is a short wide channel connecting the beginning of the left pulmonary artery with the arch of the aorta immediately distal to the origin of the left subclavian artery. It conducts most of the blood from the right ventricle into the aorta, thus shortcircuiting the lungs. After birth it is closed functionally within about a week and anatomically within about 8 weeks. The remnants of the ductus form a fibrous band called the *ligamentum arteriosum.* The left recurrent laryngeal nerve hooks around the ligamentum arteriosum.

  The ductus may remain patent after birth. The condition is called *patent ductus arteriosus* and may cause serious problems. The condition can be surgically treated.
- *Aortic aneurysm* is a localised dilatation of the aorta which may press upon the surrounding structures and cause the mediastinal syndrome, i.e. dyspnoea, dysphagia, dysphonia, etc.

20

Trachea, Oesophagus and Thoracic Duct

TRACHEA

The trachea is a wide tube lying more or less in the midline, in the lower part of the neck and in the superior mediastinum. Its upper end is continuous with the lower end of the larynx. At its lower end the trachea ends by dividing into the right and left principal bronchi.

The trachea is 10–15 cm in length. Its external diameter measures about 2 cm in males and 1.5 cm in females. The lumen is smaller in the living than in the cadaver. It is about 3 mm at one year of age. During childhood it corresponds to the age in years, with a maximum of about 12 mm in adults.

The upper end of the trachea lies at the lower border of the cricoid cartilage, opposite the sixth cervical vertebra. In the cadaver its bifurcated lower end lies at the lower border of the fourth thoracic vertebra, corresponding in front to the sternal angle (Fig. 20.1).

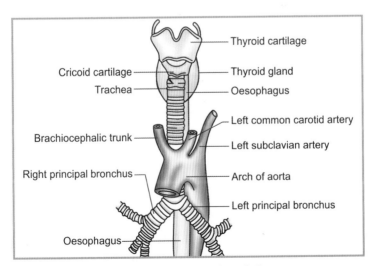

Fig. 20.1: Trachea and its relations.

151

OESOPHAGUS

The oesophagus is a narrow muscular tube, forming the food passage between the pharynx and stomach. It extends from the lower part of the neck to the upper part of the abdomen (Fig. 20.1). The oesophagus is about 25 cm long.

The oesophagus begins in the neck at the lower border of the cricoid cartilage where it is continuous with the lower end of the pharynx.

It descends in front of the vertebral column through the superior and posterior parts of the mediastinum, and pierces the diaphragm at the level of tenth thoracic vertebra. It ends by opening into the stomach at its cardiac end at the level of eleventh thoracic vertebra.

Constrictions

Normally the oesophagus shows 4 constrictions at the following levels
1. At its beginning, 15 cm from the incisor teeth
2. Where it is crossed by the aortic arch, 22.5 cm from the incisor teeth
3. Where it is crossed by the left bronchus, 27.5 cm from the incisor teeth
4. Where it pierces the diaphragm 37.5 cm from the incisor teeth

Relations of the Thoracic Part of the Oesophagus

Anterior
- (i) Trachea
- (ii) Right pulmonary artery
- (iii) Left bronchus
- (iv) Pericardium with left atrium
- (v) Diaphragm

Posteriorly
- (i) Vertebral column
- (ii) Right posterior intercostal arteries
- (iii) Thoracic duct
- (iv) Azygos vein with the terminal parts of the hemiazygos veins
- (v) Thoracic aorta
- (vi) Right pleural recess
- (vii) Diaphragm

To the right
- (i) Right lung and pleura
- (ii) Azygos vein
- (iii) The right vagus

To the left
- (i) Aortic arch
- (ii) Left subclavian artery
- (iii) Thoracic duct
- (iv) Left lung and pleura
- (v) Left recurrent laryngeal nerve, all in the superior mediastinum.

In the posterior mediastinum, it is related to:
(i) The descending thoracic aorta
(ii) The left lung and mediastinal pleura

THORACIC DUCT

The thoracic duct is the largest lymphatic vessel in the body. It extends from the upper part of the abdomen to the lower part of the neck, crossing the posterior and superior parts of the mediastinum. It is about 45 cm long. It has a beaded appearance because of the presence of many valves in its lumen.

Course

The thoracic duct begins as a continuation of the upper end of the cisterna chyli near the lower border of the twelfth thoracic vertebra and enters the thorax through the aortic opening of the diaphragm. It then ascends through the posterior mediastinum crossing from the right side to the left at the level of the fifth thoracic vertebra. It then runs through the superior mediastinum along the edge of the oesophagus and reaches the neck.

In the neck, it arches laterally at the level of the transverse process of seventh cervical vertebra. Finally it descends in front of the first part of the left subclavian artery and ends by opening into the angle of junction between the left subclavian and left internal jugular veins.

Tributaries

The thoracic duct receives lymph from, roughly, both halves of the body below the diaphragm and the left half above the diaphragm.

In the thorax, the thoracic duct receives lymph vessels from the posterior mediastinal nodes and from small intercostal nodes. At the root of the neck, efferent vessels of the nodes in the neck form the *left jugular trunk,* and those from nodes in the axilla form the *left subclavian trunk.* These trunks end either in the thoracic duct or in one of the large veins. The *left mediastinal trunk* drains lymph from the left half of the thorax, usually it ends in the brachiocephalic vein, but may end in the thoracic duct.

CLINICAL ANATOMY

- In radiographs, the trachea is seen as a vertical translucent shadow due to the contained air in front of the cervicothoracic spine.
- Clinically the trachea is palpated in the suprasternal notch. Normally it is median in position. Shift of the trachea to any side indicates a mediastinal shift.
- During swallowing when the larynx is elevated, the trachea elongates by stretching because the tracheal bifurcation is not permitted to move

by the aortic arch. Any downward pull due to sudden and forced inspiration, or aortic aneurysm will produce the physical sign known as 'tracheal tug'.

- *Tracheostomy:* It is a surgical procedure which allows air to enter directly into trachea. It is done in cases of blockage of air pathway in nose or larynx.
- As the tracheal rings are incomplete posteriorly the oesophagus can dilate during swallowing. This also allows the diameter of the trachea to be controlled by the trachealis muscle. This muscle narrows the caliber of the tube, compressing the contained air if the vocal cords are closed. This increases the explosive force of the blast of compressed air, as occurs in coughing and sneezing.
- Mucous secretions help in trapping inhaled foreign particles, and the soiled mucus is then expelled by coughing. The cilia of the mucous membrane beat upwards, pushing the mucus towards the pharynx.
- The trachea may get compressed by pathological enlargements of the thyroid, the thymus, lymph nodes and the aortic arch. This causes dyspnoea, irritative cough, and often a husky voice.
- In portal hypertension, the communications between the portal and systemic veins draining the lower end of the oesophagus dilate. These dilatations are called *oesophageal varices.* Rupture of these varices can cause serious haematemesis or vomiting of blood. The oesophageal varices can be visualised radiographically by barium swallow; they produce worm-like shadows.
- Left atrial enlargement as in mitral stenosis can also be visualised by barium swallow. The enlarged atrium causes a shallow depression on the front of the oesophagus. Barium swallow also helps in the diagnosis of oesophageal strictures, carcinoma and achalasia cardia.
- The normal indentations on the oesophagus should be kept in mind during oesophagoscopy.
- The lower end of the oesophagus is normally kept closed. It is opened by the stimulus of a food bolus. In case of neuromuscular incoordination, the lower end of the oesophagus fails to dilate with the arrival of food which, therefore, accumulates in the oesophagus. This condition of neuromuscular incoordination characterised by inability of the oesophagus to dilate is known as 'achalasia cardia'. It may be due to congenital absence of nerve cells in oesophagus.
- Improper separation of the trachea from the oesophagus during development gives rise to tracheo-oesophageal fistula.
- Compression of the oesophagus in cases of mediastinal syndrome causes dysphagia (or difficulty in swallowing).

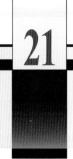

21

Surface Marking of Thorax

Surface marking is the projection of deeper structures on the surface of body.

Surface Marking of the Cardiac Valves and the Auscultatory Areas

Sound produced by closure of the valves of the heart can be heard using a stethoscope. The sound arising in relation to a particular valve are best heard not directly over the valve, but at areas situated some distance away from the valve in the direction of blood flow through it. These are called auscultatory areas. The position of the valves in relation to the surface of the body, and of the auscultatory areas is given in Table 21.1.

Table 21.1: Surface marking of the cardiac valves and the sites of the ausculatory areas

Valve	Diameter of orifice	Surface marking	Auscultatory area
1. Pulmonary	2.5 cm	A horizontal line, 2.5 cm long, behind the upper border of the third left costal cartilage and adjoining part of the sternum	Second left intercostal space near the sternum
2. Aortic	2.5 cm	A slightly oblique line, 2.5 cm long, behind the left half of the sternum at the level of the lower border of the left third costal cartilage	Second right costal cartilage near the sternum
3. Mitral	3 cm	An oblique line, 3 cm long; behind the left half of the sternum opposite the left fourth costal cartilage	Cardiac apex
4. Tricuspid	4 cm	Most oblique of all valves, being nearly vertical, 4 cm long; behind the right half of the sternum opposite the fourth and fifth spaces	Lower end of the sternum

Arteries

Internal Mammary (Thoracic) Artery

It is marked by joining the following points.

(i) A point 1 cm above the sternal end of the clavicle, 3.5 cm from the median plane

(ii) Points marked over the upper 6 costal cartilages at a distance of 1.25 cm from the lateral sternal border

(iii) The last point is marked in the sixth space 1.25 cm from the lateral sternal border

Arch of the Aorta

Arch of the aorta lies behind the lower half of the manubrium sterni. Its upper convex border is marked by a line which begins at the right end of the sternal angle, arches upwards and to the left through the centre of the manubrium, and ends at the sternal end of the left second costal cartilage. Note that the beginning and the end of the arch lie at the same level. When marked on the surface as described above the arch looks much smaller than it actually is because of foreshortening.

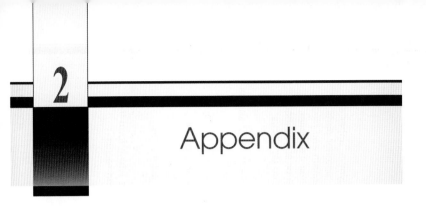

2

Appendix

Appendix 2 at the end of the section on thorax gives a bird's eye view of the sympathetic component of the autonomic nervous system. The course of the typical and atypical intercostal nerves is also mentioned. Arteries of thorax have been tabulated in Tables A2.1 and A.2.2. Various clinical terms are defined.

AUTONOMIC NERVOUS SYSTEM

The autonomic nervous system comprises sympathetic and parasympathetic components. Sympathetic is active during fright, flight or fight. During any of these activities, the pupils dilate, skin gets pale, blood pressure rises, blood vessels of skeletal muscles, heart, lungs and brain dilate. There is hardly any activity in the digestive tracts due to which the individual does not feel hungry. The person is tense and gets tired soon.

Parasympathetic has the opposite effects of sympathetic. This component is sympathetic to the digestive tract. In its activity digestion and metabolism of food occurs. Heart beats normally. Person is relaxed and can do creative work. Autonomic nervous system is controlled by brainstem and cerebral hemispheres. These include reticular formation of brainstem, thalamic and hypothalamic nuclei, limbic lobe and prefrontal cortex including the ascending and descending tracts interconnecting these regions.

Sympathetic Nervous System

Sympathetic nervous system is the larger of the two components of autonomic nervous system. It consists of two ganglionated trunks, their branches, prevertebral ganglia, plexuses. It supplies all the viscera of thorax, abdomen and pelvis, including the blood vessels of head and neck, brain, limbs, skin and the sweat glands as well as arrector pilorum muscle of skin.

The preganglionic fibres are the axons of neurons situated in the lateral horns of T1–L2 segments of spinal cord. They leave spinal cord through

Table A2.1: Arteries of thorax

Artery	Origin, course and termination	Area of distribution
Internal thoracic	Arises from inferior aspect of 1st part of subclavian artery. Its origin lies 2 cm above the sternal end of the clavicle. It runs onwards, forwards and medially behind the clavicle and behind the 1–6 costal cartilages and 1–5 intercostal spaces to terminate in the 6th intercostal space by dividing into superior epigastric and musculophrenic arteries	It supplies pericardium, thymus, upper six intercostal spaces in their anterior parts, mammary gland, rectus sheath and also 7–9 intercostal spaces. Thus it supplies anterior thoracic and anterior abdominal walls from the clavicle to the umbilicus
Pericardiophrenic artery	Branch of internal thoracic artery	Supplies fibrous and parietal layer of serous pericardia and the diaphragm
Mediastinal arteries	Small branches of internal thoracic artery	Supply thymus and fat in the mediastinum
Two anterior intercostal arteries	Two arteries each arise in 1–6 upper intercostal spaces from internal thoracic.	Supply muscles of the 1–6 intercostal spaces and parietal pleura
Perforating arteries	Arise from internal thoracic artery in 2nd, 3rd and 4th spaces	They are large enough to supply the mammary gland
Superior epigastric artery	Terminal branch of internal thoracic artery. Enters the rectus sheath and ends by anastomosing with inferior epigastric A, a branch of external iliac artery	Supplies the aponeuroses which form the rectus sheath, including the rectus abdominis.
Musculophrenic artery	This is also the terminal branch of internal thoracic artery. Ends by giving 2 anterior intercostal arteries in 7–9 intercostal spaces and by supplying the thoraco-abdominal diaphragm	Supplies the muscles of anterior parts of 7–9 intercostal spaces, and the muscle fibres of the thoracoabdominal diaphragm

(Contd.)

Table A2.1: Arteries of thorax *(Contd.)*

Artery	Origin, course and termination	Area of distribution
Ascending aorta	Arise from the upper end of left ventricle. It is about 5 cm long and is enclosed in the pericardium. It runs upwards, forwards and to the right and continues as the arch of aorta at the sternal end of upper border of 2nd right costal cartilage. At the root of aorta, there are three dilatations of the vessel wall called the aortic sinuses. These are anterior, left posterior and right posterior	Supplies the heart musculature with the help of right coronary and left coronary arteries, described later.
Arch of aorta	It begins behind the upper border of 2nd right sterno-chondral joint. Runs upwards, backwards and to left across the left side of bifurcation of trachea. Then it passes behind the left bronchus and on the left side of of body of T4 vertebra by becoming continuous with the descending thoracic aorta	Through its three branches namely brachio-cephalic, left common carotid and left subclavian arteries, arch of aorta supplies part of brain, head, neck and upper limb
Brachiocephalic trunk	1st branch of arch of aorta. Runs upwards and soon divides into right common carotid and right subclavian arteries.	Through these two branches part of the right half of brain, head, neck are supplied. The distribution of 2 branches on right side is same as on the left side
Left common carotid artery	It runs upwards on the left side of trachea and at upper border of thyroid cartilage. The artery ends by dividing into internal carotid and external carotid arteries	The two branches supply brain, structures in the head and neck
Left subclavian artery	It is the last branch of arch of aorta. Runs to left in the root of neck behind scalenus anterior muscle, then on the upper surface of 1st rib. At the outer border of 1st rib, it continues as the axillary artery	Gives branches which supply part of brain, part of thyroid gland, muscles around scapula, 1st and 2nd posterior intercostal spaces

(Contd.)

Table A2.1: Arteries of thorax (Contd.)

Artery	Origin, course and termination	Area of distribution
Descending thoracic aorta	Begins on the left side of the lower border of body of T4 vertebra. Descends with inclination to right and ends at the lower border of T12 vertebra by continuing as abdominal aorta	3–11 posterior intercostal spaces, subcostal area, lung tissue, oesophagus, pericardium, mediastinum and diaphragm
3–11 posterior intercostal arteries	3–11 posterior intercostal arteries of both right and left sides arise from the descending thoracic aorta. Right branches are little longer than the left. Each intercostal artery and its collateral branch end by anastomosing with the two anterior intercostal arteries	Supply the muscles of these intercostal spaces. Each of these arteries gives a collateral branch, which runs along the lower border of the respective intercostal space
Bronchial arteries	Two left bronchial arteries arise from descending aorta	Bronchial tree
Oesophageal branches	2–3 oesophageal branches arise from descending aorta.	Supply the oesophagus
Pericardial branches	Branches of descending aorta, run on the pericardium	Fibrous and parietal layer of serous pericardia.
Mediastinal branches	Arise from descending aorta.	Supply lymph nodes and fat in posterior mediastinum.
Superior phrenic arteries	Two branches of descending aorta. End in the superior surface of diaphragm. These arteries anastomose with branches of musculophrenic and pericardiophrenic arteries.	Supply the thoracoabdominal diaphragm

Table A2.2: Comparison of right and left coronary arteries

Right coronary artery	Left coronary artery
1. Origin: Anterior aortic sinus of ascending aorta	1. Left posterior aortic sinus of ascending aorta
2. Course: Between pulmonary trunk and right auricle	2. Between pulmonary trunk and left auricle
3. Descends in atrioventricular groove on the right side	3. Descends in atrioventricular groove on the left side
4. Turns at the inferior border to run in posterior part of atrioventricular groove	4. Turns at left border to run in posterior part of atrioventricular groove. It is now called as circumflex branch
5. Termination: Ends by anastomosing with the circumflex branch of left coronary artery	5. Its circumflex branch ends by anastomosing with right coronary artery
6. Branches: To right atrium, right ventricle (marginal artery) and posterior interventricular branch for both ventricles and interventricular septa	6. Left atrium, left ventricle and anterior interventricular branch for both ventricles and interventricular septa. Anterior interventricular branch ends by anastomosing with posterior interventricular branch

their respective ventral roots, to pass in their nerve trunks, and beginning of ventral rami via white ramus communicans (WRC). There are 14 WRC on each side. These fibres can have following alternative routes.

(i) They relay in the ganglion of the sympathetic trunks, postganglionic fibres pass via the grey communicans and get distributed to the blood vessels of muscles, skin, sweat glands and to arrector pili muscles.

(ii) These may pass through the corresponding ganglion and ascend to a ganglion higher before terminating in the above manner.

(iii) These may pass through the corresponding ganglion and descend to a ganglion lower and then terminate in the above manner.

(iv) These may synapse in the corresponding ganglia and pass medially to the viscera like heart, lungs, oesophagus.

(v) These white rami communicans pass to corresponding ganglia and emerge from these as WRC (unrelayed) in the form of splanchnic nerves to supply abdominal and pelvic viscera after synapsing in the ganglia situated in the abdominal cavity. Some fibres of splanchnic nerves pass express to *adrenal medulla*.

Sympathetic trunk on either side of the body extends from cervical region to the coccygeal region where both trunks fuse to form a single *ganglion impar*. It has cervical, thoracic, lumbar, sacral and coccygeal parts.

Thoracic Part of Sympathetic Trunk

There are usually 11 ganglia on the sympathetic trunk of thoracic part. The first ganglion lies on neck of Ist rib and is usually fused with inferior cervical ganglion and forms stellate ganglion. The lower ones lie on the heads of the ribs. The sympathetic trunk continues with its abdominal part by passing behind the medial arcuate ligament.

The ganglia are connected with the respective spinal nerves via the white ramus communicans (from the spinal nerve to the ganglion) and the grey ramus communicans (from the ganglion to the spinal nerve, i.e. ganglion gives grey).

Branches

1. Grey rami communicans to all the spinal nerves, i.e. T1–T12. The postganglionic fibres pass along the spinal nerves to supply cutaneous blood vessels, sweat glands and arrector pili muscles.
2. White rami communicans from T1–T6 ganglia travel up to the cervical part of sympathetic trunk to relay in the three cervical ganglia. Fibres from the lower thoracic ganglia T10–L2 pass down as preganglionic fibres to relay in the lumbar or sacral ganglia.
3. The first five ganglia give postganglionic fibres to heart, lungs, aorta and oesophagus.
4. Lower eight ganglia give fibres which are preganglionic (unrelayed) for the supply of abdominal viscera. These are called as splanchnic (visceral) nerves.

Table A2.3: Components of deep cardiac plexus

Right half	Left half
1. Superior, middle, inferior cervical cardiac branches of right sympathetic trunk	Only middle and inferior branches
2. Cardiac branches of T2–T4 ganglia of right side	Same
3. Superior and inferior cervical cardiac branches of right vagus	Only the superior cervical cardiac branch of left vagus
4. Thoracic cardiac branch of right vagus	Same
5. Two branches of right recurrent laryngeal nerve arising from neck region	Same, but coming from thoracic region

Ganglia 5–9 give fibres which constitute greater splanchnic nerve. Some fibres reach adrenal medulla.

Ganglia 9–10 give fibres that constitute lesser splanchnic nerve.

Ganglion 11 gives fibres that constitute lowest splanchnic nerve.

Nerve Supply of Heart

Preganglionic sympathetic neurons are located in lateral horns T1–T5 segments of spinal cord. These fibres pass along the respective ventral roots of thoracic nerves, to synapse with the respective ganglia of the sympathetic trunk. After relay the postganglionic fibres form thoracic branches which intermingle with the vagal fibres, to form cardiac plexus.

Some fibres from T1–T5 segments of spinal cord reach their respective ganglia. These fibres then travel up to the cervical part of the sympathetic chain and relay in superior, middle and inferior cervical ganglia. After relay, the postganglionic fibres form the three cervical cardiac nerves. Preganglionic parasympathetic neurons for the supply of heart are situated in the dorsal nucleus of vagus nerve.

Sympathetic activity increases the heart rate. Larger branches of coronary are mainly supplied by sympathetic. It causes vasodilatation of coronary arteries. Impulses of pain travel along sympathetic fibres. These fibres pass mostly through left sympathetic trunk and reach the spinal cord via T1–T5 spinal nerves. Thus the pain may be referred to the area of skin supplied by T1–T5 nerves, i.e. retrosternal, medial side of the upper limbs. Since one is more conscious of impulses coming from skin than the viscera one feels as if the pain is in the skin. This is the basis of the referred pain.

Smaller branches of coronary artery are supplied by parasympathetic nerves. These nerves are concerned with slowing of the cardiac cycle.

The nerves reach the heart by the following two plexuses.

Superficial Cardiac Plexus

Superficial cardiac plexus is formed by the following
  (i) Superior cervical cardiac branch of left sympathetic trunk
 (ii) Inferior cervical cardiac branch of left vagus nerve

Deep Cardiac Plexus

Deep cardiac plexus consists of two halves which are interconnected and lie anterior to bifurcation of trachea (Table A2.3).

Branches from the cardiac plexus give extensive branches to pulmonary plexuses, right and left coronary plexuses. Branches from the coronary plexuses supply both the atria and the ventricles. Left ventricle gets richer nerve supply because of its larger size.

Nerve Supply of Lungs

The lungs are supplied from the anterior and posterior pulmonary plexuses. Anterior plexus is an extension of deep cardiac plexus. The posterior is formed from branches of vagus and T2–T5 sympathetic ganglia. Small ganglia are found on these nerves for the relay of parasympathetic brought via vagal nerve fibres. Parasympathetic is broncho-constrictor or motor whereas sympathetic is inhibitory. Sympathetic stimulation causes relaxation of smooth muscles of bronchial tubes or bronchodilator. The pressure of inspired air also causes bronchodilatation.

TYPICAL INTERCOSTAL NERVE

Typical intercostal nerves are any of the nerves belonging to 3rd to 6th intercostal spaces.

Beginning

Typical thoracic spinal nerve after it has given off dorsal primary ramus or dorsal ramus is called the intercostal nerve. It runs in the intercostal space, i.e. between the lower border of rib above and upper border of rib below.

Course

Typical intercostal nerve enters the posterior part of intercostal space by passing behind the posterior intercostal vessels. So the intercostal nerve lies lowest in the neurovascular bundle. The order from above downwards is vein, artery and nerve (VAN). At first the bundle runs between posterior intercostal membrane and subcostalis, then between internal intercostal and innermost intercostal and lastly between internal intercostal and sternocostalis muscles.

At the anterior end of intercostal space, the intercostal nerve passes in front of internal thoracic vessels, pierces internal intercostal muscle and anterior intercostal membrane to continue as anterior cutaneous branch which ends by dividing into medial and lateral cutaneous branches.

Branches

1. Communicating branches to the sympathetic ganglion close to the beginning of ventral ramus. The anterior ramus containing sympathetic fibres from lateral horn of spinal cord gives off a *white ramus communicans* to the sympathetic ganglion. These fibres get relayed in the ganglion. Some of these relayed fibres pass via *grey ramus communicans* to ventral ramus. Few pass backwards in the dorsal ramus and rest pass through the ventral ramus. These sympathetic fibres are sudomotor, pilomotor and vasomotor to the skin and vasodilator to the skeletal vessels.

2. Before the angle, nerve gives a collateral branch that runs along the upper border of lower rib. This branch supplies intercostal muscles, costal pleura and periosteum of the rib.
3. Lateral cutaneous branch arises along the midaxillary line. It divides into anterior and posterior branches.
4. The nerve keeps giving muscular, periosteal and branches to the costal pleura during its course.
5. Anterior cutaneous branch is the terminal branch of the nerve.

ATYPICAL INTERCOSTAL NERVES

The thoracic spinal nerves which do not follow absolutely thoracic course are designated as atypical intercostal nerves. Thus intercostal one, two, are atypical as these two nerves partly supply the upper limb.

The first thoracic nerve entirely joins the brachial plexus as its last rami or root. It gives no contribution to the first intercostal space. That is why the nerve supply of skin of first intercostal space is from the supraclavicular nerves (C3, C4).

The second thoracic or second intercostal nerve runs in the second intercostal space. But its lateral cutaneous branch as intercostobrachial nerve is rather big and it supplies skin of the axilla as well. Third to sixth intercostal nerves are typical.

Also seventh, eighth, ninth, tenth, eleventh intercostal nerves are atypical, as these course partly through thoracic wall and partly through antero-lateral abdominal wall. Lastly the twelfth thoracic is known as subcostal nerve. It also passes through the anterolateral abdominal muscles. These nerves supply, parietal peritoneum, muscles and overlying skin.

CLINICAL ANATOMY

Site of pericardial tapping: Removal of pericardial fluid is done in left *4th or 5th intercostal* spaces just left of the sternum as pleura deviates exposing the pericardium against the medial part of left 4th and 5th intercostal spaces. Care should be taken to avoid injury to internal thoracic artery lying at a distance of 1 cm from the lateral border of sternum. Needle can also be passed upwards and posteriorly from the left xiphicostal angle to reach the pericardial cavity.

Foreign bodies in trachea: Foreign bodies like pins, coins entering the trachea pass into right bronchus; Right bronchus wider, more vertical and is in line with trachea. Most of the human beings want to take the path of least resistance, so the foreign bodies in the trachea travel down into right bronchus and then into posterior basal segments of the lower lobe of the lung.

Site of bone marrow puncture: The manubrium sterni is the favoured site for bone *marrow puncture* in adults. Manubrium is subcutaneous and easily approachable. Bone marrow studies are done for various haematological disorders. Another site is the iliac crest; which is the preferred site in children.

Posture of a patient with respiratory difficulty: Such a patient finds comfort while sitting, as diaphragm is lowest in this position. In lying position, the diaphragm is highest and patient is very uncomfortable.

In standing position, the diaphragm level is midway, but the patient is too sick to stand.

Patient also fixes the arms by holding the arms of a chair, so that serratus anterior and pectoralis major can move the ribs and help in respiration.

Paracentesis thoracis or pleural tapping: Aspiration of any fluid from the pleural cavity is called *paracentesis thoracis*. It is usually done in the eighth intercostal space in midaxillary line. The needle is passed through lower part of space to avoid injury to the principal neurovascular bundle.

Some clinical conditions associated with the pleura are as follows.

Pleurisy: This is inflammation of the pleura. It may be dry, but often it is accompanied by collection of fluid in the pleural cavity. The condition is called the pleural effusion.

Pneumothorax: Presence of air in the pleural cavity.

Haemothorax: Presence of blood in the pleural cavity.

Hydropneumothorax: Presence of both fluid and air in the pleural cavity.

Empyema: Presence of pus in the pleural cavity.

Coronary artery: Thrombosis of a coronary artery is a common cause of sudden death in persons past middle age. This is due to myocardial infarction and ventricular fibrillation.

Incomplete obstruction, usually due to spasm of the coronary artery causes angina pectoris, which is associated with agonising pain in the precordial region and down the medial side of the left arm and forearm.

Coronary angiography determines the site(s) of narrowing or occlusion of the coronary arteries or their branches.

Angioplasty helps in removal of small block age. It is done using small stent or small inflated balloon.

If there are large segments or multiple sites of blockage, coronary bypass is done using either great saphenous vein or internal thoracic artery as graft(s).

Cardiac pain is an ischaemic pain caused by incomplete obstruction of a coronary artery.

Axons of pain fibres conveyed by the sensory sympathetic cardiac nerves reach thoracic one to thoracic five segments of spinal cord mostly through the dorsal root ganglia of the left side. These dorsal root ganglia also receive sensory impulses from the medial side of arm, forearm and upper part of front of chest.

Though the pain is usually referred to the left side, it may even be referred to right arm, jaw, epigastrium or back.

Oesophageal varices: In portal hypertension, the communications between the portal and systemic veins draining the lower end of the oesophagus dilate. These dilatations are called *oesophageal varices.* Rupture of these varices can cause serious haematemesis or vomiting of blood. The oesophageal varices can be visualised radiographically by barium swallow; they produce worm-like shadows.

Barium swallow: Left atrial enlargement as in mitral stenosis can also be visualised by barium swallow. The enlarged atrium causes a shallow depression on the front of the oesophagus. Barium swallow also helps in the diagnosis of oesophageal strictures, carcinoma and achalasia cardia.

Coarctation of the aorta: Coarctation of the aorta is a localised narrowing of the aorta opposite to or just beyond the attachment of the ductus arteriosus. An extensive collateral circulation develops between the branches of the subclavian arteries and those of the descending aorta. These include the anastomoses between the anterior and posterior intercostal arteries. These arteries enlarge greatly and produce a characteristic notching on the ribs.

Aortic aneurysm: Aortic aneurysm is a localised dilatation of the aorta which may press upon the surrounding structures and cause the mediastinal syndrome.

Index

Aperture of thorax
   inferior 103
   superior 101
Apex of the heart 138
Arch of aorta 148, 156
Arm 46
Arteries
   of thorax
      arch of aorta 159
      ascending aorta 159
      brachiocephalic 159
      broncheal 160
      coronary arteries 161
      descending thoracic/aorta 160
      internal thoracic 158
Autonomic nervous system 157
Axilla 26, 31

Back 32
Bones
   of thorax 105
      ribs 105
      sternum 109
      vertebral column 111
   of upper limb 5
      carpal bones 12
      clavicle 5
      humerus 8
      metacarpals 14
      phalanges 15
      radius 10
      scapula 6
      ulna 11
Brachial plexus 27
Breast/mammary gland 19
   lymphatic drainage 20
   self-examination 25
Bronchial tree 129
Bronchopulmonary
   segments 129

Cardiac pain 120, 147
Cardiac valves 155
Carpel tunnel syndrome 96
Cervical rib 104
Clinical terms
   thorax 165
   upper limb 91
Compartments of arm 46
Conducting system of
   heart 143
Coronary bypass 146
Cubital fossa 48
Cubital tunnel syndrome 96

Deep cardiac plexus 163
Deep palmar arch 83
Dermatomes 35, 38

Erb's paralysis 29
Eye of the hand 65

Flexer retinaculum 52, 83

Ganglion impar 162
Golfer's elbow 96

Heart 138
   left atrium 142
   left ventricle 142
   nerve supply 163
   right atrium 139
   right ventricle 141
   surfaces 139
   valves 143

Intravenous infection 97
   clinical anatomy
   of thorax
      and pleura 121
      and thoracic duct 153
      aorta and pulmonary

bones and joints 116
heart 136
introduction 104
lungs 131
mediastinum 134
pericardium and
superior vena cava,
thoracic cavity
trachea, oesophagus
trunk 150
of upper limb
arm 51
axilla 29
bones 16
dermatomes and
forearm and hand 62
joints 78
pectoral region 24
scapular region 44
superficial veins 38

Joints
of thorax 114
of upper limb
elbow 71
of hand 77
radioulnar 73
shoulder girdle 68
shoulder joint 70
wrist 75
Klumpke's paralysis 30

Labourer's nerve 62
Lungs 125
fissures and lobes 126
nerve supply 164
root 126
Lymphadenitis 39
Lymphangitis 39

Mammogram 25
Mediastinum 132
inferior 133
superior 133
Muscles
connecting upper limb
to vertebral column 33
intercostal muscles 118

of pectoral region 23
of scapular column 41
deltoid 40
of arm 47
of back of forearm 63, 64
of forearm 53, 56
of hand 57
serratus anterior 22
triceps brachii 50
Musician's nerve 66

Nerves
of upper limb
axillary 86
median 87
musculocutaneous 48, 85
radial 51, 86
ulnar 88
of thorax
atypical intercostal 165
typical intercostal 164

Oesophagus 152

Parts of upper limb 3
Pericardium
fibrous 136
serous 137
sinuses 137
Pleura 121
Precordium 146
Pulse 62

Quadrangular space 43

Respiratory movements 116
Retinacula
extensor 55, 83
flexer 52, 83
Ribs 105
Rotator cuff 43

Space
lower triangular 44
midpalmar 60
of hand 55
quadrangular 43
thenar 60
upper triangular 44

Surface marking
   of thorax 155
   of thorax limb 82
Sympathetic nervous
   system 157
Thoracic duct 153
Trachea 151

Vein
Vertebral column 111
   basilic 37
cephalic 37
dorsal venous arch 36
median cubital 37
of upper limb 36
superficial veins
   of upper limb 36

Waiter's tip 96
Walls of thorax 118
Wrist drop 51, 96

Xiphoid process 110